PRAISE FOR
RECOVERY ALLIES

"Given the unrelenting and increasing burden of disease, disability, and premature mortality caused by addiction, Alison Jones Webb highlights an undeniable social reality—that if we're serious about addressing the addiction crisis, we need to get on the same page, unite, and work together to stand any real chance of making a meaningful and lasting difference. Webb has done a great service at a time of national crisis through expansive review and her articulate, easily digestible summary of the new science of addiction recovery. This book should inspire and empower policy makers and the public alike to become 'allies in recovery.'"

—JOHN F. KELLY, PhD, ABPP, Elizabeth R. Spallin
Professor of Psychiatry in Addiction Medicine at
Harvard Medical School and founder and director
of the Recovery Research Institute, Massachusetts
General Hospital

"This is the resource I will be pointing everyone to when they ask how they can help someone with substance use disorder. The right response is always 'educate yourself!'—and this book helps people do just that. Alison Jones Webb compassionately articulates a complex, complicated topic and provides actionable steps that anyone can do. Nonclinical language makes the book very accessible, as the author carefully unravels some of the causes and conditions around trauma and mental health with personal stories, expanding the perspective of what recovery looks like. Webb shines a bright light on the many benefits offered by the recovery community. I'm excited to share this book with our readers."

—CAROLYN DELANEY, founder and publisher of
Journey magazine and person in long-term recovery

"Finally, a book with solutions to our national addiction epidemic—I hope allies and decision makers pay close attention! Simply a wonderful book, a godsend. One of the best books of its kind I've ever read."

—JOHN SHINHOLSER, president of The McShin
Foundation and person in long-term recovery

"Alison Jones Webb has made an excellent contribution to the growing literature on addiction recovery. *Recovery Allies* is based on strong research evidence and a wonderfully diverse set of interviews with many key figures in the recovery research and practice field. This book is clear and concise and makes a compelling addition to our understanding of the key role communities and social networks play in the complex pathways to addiction recovery."

—DAVID BEST, PhD, professor of criminology at the University of Derby and author of *Pathways to Recovery and Desistance*

"If you know of a loved one, friend, coworker, or neighbor—really any human being—struggling with substance use disorder but don't know how to help them, this book will explain how to be an ally and give the support that might just save a life. I wish I had had the knowledge contained in this book during my law enforcement career and when I realized my daughter was struggling with an opioid use disorder. It would have changed my approach and made a positive difference."

—BOB MACKENZIE, chief of police, Kennebunk, Maine, and affected family member

"This is an important book, one that I could have used when trying to support my nephew's ongoing struggle with opioid addiction. Tragically, we lost him to an overdose in 2018. This wonderful, well-researched book comes too late for our family, but I have great hope that it will help many others avoid this terrible and avoidable outcome."

—LISA HALLEE, JD, CPCC (Certified Professional Co-Active Coach) and affected family member

"Alison Jones Webb courageously tackles the root causes of substance use disorder, including trauma and mental health, and thoughtfully explores the barriers encountered by those in recovery, most especially shame and stigma. She provides readers with practical and authentic approaches to creating a recovery-friendly community. This book is an essential read for those serving and interacting with individuals in recovery and for those who want to make a difference in their communities."

—DR. ALANE O'CONNOR, DNP, clinical advisor at MaineMOM (Maine Maternal Opioid Misuse)

RECOVERY
ALLIES

How to Support
Addiction Recovery
and Build Recovery-Friendly
Communities

ALISON JONES WEBB, MA, MPH
FOREWORD BY PHILLIP VALENTINE

North Atlantic Books
Huichin, unceded Ohlone land
aka Berkeley, California

Figure 1.4, "Stages of Change and Related Treatment and Recovery Support Services" adapted with permission from the Recovery Research Institute, Massachusetts General Hospital.

"Recovery Capital Scale" reprinted with permission from William L. White.

Published by   Cover art © turtleteeth via Shutterstock.com
North Atlantic Books   Cover design by Mimi Bark
Huichin, unceded Ohlone land   Book design by Happenstance Type-O-Rama
aka Berkeley, California

Printed in the United States of America

Recovery Allies: How to Support Addiction Recovery and Build Recovery-Friendly Communities is sponsored and published by North Atlantic Books, an educational nonprofit based in the unceded Ohlone land Huichin (*aka* Berkeley, CA) that collaborates with partners to develop cross-cultural perspectives; nurture holistic views of art, science, the humanities, and healing; and seed personal and global transformation by publishing work on the relationship of body, spirit, and nature.

MEDICAL DISCLAIMER: The following information is intended for general information purposes only. Individuals should always see their health care provider before administering any suggestions made in this book. Any application of the material set forth in the following pages is at the reader's discretion and is their sole responsibility.

North Atlantic Books' publications are distributed to the US trade and internationally by Penguin Random House Publisher Services. For further information, visit our website at www.northatlanticbooks.com.

Library of Congress Cataloging-in-Publication Data

Names: Webb, Alison Jones, author.
Title: Recovery allies : how to support addiction recovery and build
   recovery-friendly communities / Alison Jones Webb.
Description: Berkeley, California : North Atlantic Books, [2022] | Includes
   bibliographical references and index. | Summary: "A practical, hopeful,
   and research-based guide for supporting loved ones through addiction and
   recovery"—Provided by publisher.
Identifiers: LCCN 2022013832 (print) | LCCN 2022013833 (ebook) | ISBN
   9781623175887 (trade paperback) | ISBN 9781623175894 (ebook)
Subjects: LCSH: Addicts—Rehabilitation. | Recovering addicts—Services
   for.
Classification: LCC HV4998 .W43 2022 (print) | LCC HV4998 (ebook) | DDC
   362.29—dc23/eng/20220404
LC record available at https://lccn.loc.gov/2022013832
LC ebook record available at https://lccn.loc.gov/2022013833

1 2 3 4 5 6 7 8 9 KPC 26 25 24 23 22

This book includes recycled material and material from well-managed forests. North Atlantic Books is committed to the protection of our environment. We print on recycled paper whenever possible and partner with printers who strive to use environmentally responsible practices.

For Jim

ACKNOWLEDGMENTS

I wrote *Recovery Allies* mostly in isolation in 2021–22 in Portland, Maine, and Charlottesville, Virginia, while the country was in a state of major upheaval. The relentless, deadly spread of COVID-19. The Black Lives Matter response to police violence. Political unrest resulting from the storming of the U.S. Capitol. An unprecedented surge in opioid overdose deaths. Calls on the left to defund the police and end the war on drugs and on the right to upend our democracy. Even with this backdrop, I felt confident envisioning a world where we all participate in creating our future together and writing about hope and social change in our communities. That's because, beyond all the data and research I had acquired, I'd seen enough true transformations in people to know that there is always—*always*—hope for healing and for situations to improve.

This book calls for collective action and individual changes of heart to create recovery-friendly communities. It's about supporting our friends, neighbors, and loved ones in recovery, but its message is more significant than that. It's about supporting each other on our chosen paths. With that in mind, I want to thank the people who made this book happen. First, I owe a tremendous debt to Anna Black for our many conversations about addiction and recovery, and her believing in creative approaches to supporting young people in recovery. She led the federally funded Substance Abuse Treatment Enhancement and Dissemination project that developed effective treatment for young adults in Maine. I'm also indebted to that project's first interns, Andrew Kiezulas, Bryn Gallagher, Alex Klein, and Matthew Braun, for their willingness to share everything they knew about recovery, and for connecting me with Portland, Maine's recovery community. They bravely paved the way for others in recovery to tell their stories. I am grateful to the staff and board of the Maine Association of Recovery Residences for the many discussions about safe recovery housing we've had during my tenure as president of the board.

The people who shared their stories in focus groups and interviews for this book and for articles in *Journey Magazine* form the backbone of discussions on what I refer to as the pillars of recovery. I spoke with Sarah Coupe, Niki Curtis, Faye Davis, Carolyn Delaney, Justin Downie, Sarah Farrugia, Cynthia Geer, Samantha Genest, Todd and Mary Grove, Tyler Hall, Erik Jones, Kayla Kalel, Tammy Kalel, Mike Kelly, Kim LaMontagne, Josh Leonard, Honesty Liller, Kaitlin MacKenzie, Michael Mihailos, LaTeefe Pele, Christopher Poulos, Danielle Rideout, Sarah Siegel, Ronald Springel, and Karen and Eddie Walsh. Four people I interviewed asked me not to publish their names, and all focus group participants were anonymous. I'm also grateful to members of my family who shared their experiences of addiction and recovery.

Other allies and recovery champions I have spoken with over the course of writing—Joanne Arnold, Jen Dean, Allen Ewing-Merrill, Jane Field, Susan Gross, Lisa Hallee, John Kilbride, Carolyn Lambert, Michael Lyon, Karen MacKenzie, Robert MacKenzie, Robbie Moulton, Liz Blackwell-Moore, Bradford Paige, Jennifer Radel, Alicia Smith, Liz Torrance, Charlotte Warren, and others—added valuable content to this book.

Professionals I interviewed who offered their wisdom and knowledge contributed significantly to discussions about evidence-based recovery support services and advocacy: John Buro, president, Portland Recovery Community Center; Tom Coderre, acting deputy assistant secretary for Mental Health and Substance Use, Substance Abuse and Mental Health Services Administration; Mary Drew, founder and chief executive officer, Reality Check; Dr. Jonathan Fellers, medical director, Crossroads Maine; Ryan Hampton, activist and founder of the Recovery Advocacy Project and author of *Unsettled: How the Purdue Pharma Bankruptcy Failed the Victims of the American Overdose Crisis;* Dr. Haner Hernández, consultant to the New England Addiction Technology Transfer Center at Brown University and to the National Latino and Hispanic ATTC; Dr. Keith Humphreys, Esther Ting Memorial Professor, Stanford University; Piers Kaniuka, chief executive officer of programming, Rockland Recovery Treatment Centers, and founder, Resistance Recovery; Dr. John Kelly, Elizabeth

R. Spallin Professor of Psychiatry in Addiction Medicine at Harvard Medical School and founder and director of the Recovery Research Institute, Massachusetts General Hospital; Dean LeMire, Recovery Support Services director, RecoveryLink; Dr. Merideth Norris, addiction physician of CAP Quality Care; Dr. Alane O'Connor, clinical advisor to the Maine Maternal Opioid Misuse Initiative and cochair of Maine's Opioid Response Clinical Advisory Committee; Philip Rutherford, chief operating officer, Faces and Voices of Recovery; David Sheridan, executive director, National Alliance for Recovery Residences; John Shinholser, co-founder and president, The McShin Foundation; Gordon Smith, Maine's director of Opioid Response; Dr. Jeffrey Spiegel, medical director and founder, Casco Bay Medical; Dr. Ronald Springel, executive director, Maine Association of Recovery Residences; Dr. Christine Timko, clinical professor, Stanford University; Phillip Valentine, executive director, Connecticut Community for Addiction Recovery; Margo Walsh, founder and chief executive officer, MaineWorks; William White, emeritus senior research consultant, Chestnut Health Systems; and Greg Williams, managing director, Third Horizon Strategies, and manager, the Alliance for Addiction Payment Reform.

Colleagues and friends at organizations too numerous to mention created safe places to talk about addiction and recovery, lifted me when spirits were low, and continue to do the day-to-day work of building recovery-friendly communities. These organizations include AdCare Educational Institute of Maine, Choose to Be Healthy Coalition, Co-Occurring Collaborative Serving Maine, The Family Restored, Health Equity Alliance of Maine, *Journey Magazine,* Maine Access Points, Maine Association of Recovery Residences, Maine-General Medical Center, Maine Recovery Advocacy Project, The McShin Foundation, Milestone Recovery, Pine Tree Recovery Center, the Portland Needle Exchange Program and Portland Public Health Division, Portland Recovery Community Center and other recovery community centers in Maine, the Recovery Oriented Campus Center at the University of Southern Maine, and Young People in Recovery.

Three people deserve special mention. First, Andrew Kiezulas has been a constant source of inspiration, knowledge, humor, and support from the beginning of my journey in the recovery world. Second, Carolyn Delaney, founder and publisher of *Journey Magazine,* has opened her doors and her heart to teach me about healing and support my recovery writing. Finally,

Patty McCarthy, friend and editor, improved the manuscript with her attention to detail and way with words, and our many conversations about addiction, recovery, and life have been deeply enriching.

I thank the team at North Atlantic Books that made my dream a reality. Keith Donnell, acquisitions associate and editor, believed in my idea, gave kind encouragement and direction, and helped see this book through to publication.

And last but certainly not least, thanks to my husband Jim, who kept the household running while I wrote this book through COVID restrictions, family illness, our son's wedding, the birth of our granddaughter, and three interstate moves. He's been my coach, critic, editor, and sounding board. Without his limitless patience, droll sense of humor, and unwavering support over thirty-eight years together, *Recovery Allies* might very well still be just a great idea instead of being here on paper.

CONTENTS

FOREWORD

I can think of no greater cause, or ambitious project, than Alison's book, *Recovery Allies,* on how to create recovery-friendly communities. Indeed, promoting recovery has been my life's work since 1999, and I personally appreciate Alison's transparency and, particularly, her unique perspective. She describes the essence of recovery succinctly, beautifully, and emotionally.

As I read, I became enamored with Alison's in-depth research and her findings. Relying on the perspective of many individuals, she encapsulates and condenses her findings in a way that is easy to read. I wholeheartedly agree with her premise that if people understand recovery, they are more likely to support recovery. And if we understand it, we are more likely to build recovery-friendly communities.

The first barrier in our way is shame and stigma. Alison shares what she uncovered. Personally, I worked through the shame of my own addiction to alcohol and cocaine. At the Connecticut Community for Addiction Recovery (CCAR), where I've worked since 1999, we abandoned the term "stigma." We believe every time we use the word "stigma," we reinforce it. As a recovery ally, I live in the solution. I believe it's far better to promote recovery than to try to reduce the stigma.

To my knowledge, this is the first book that provides specific advocacy tools and discusses overarching public health strategies while underscoring the prominent role of personal connection as essential to personal recovery. The thread of connection weaves its way through every chapter of *Recovery Allies.* Look for it. Reflect on how connection plays a role in your life. Look for the connective tissue in your local community. Can you find it? What *is* that connection?

After many, many years of facilitating training for recovery coaches, I believe that connection consists mostly of love. Yes, I used the "L" word!

While addicted, I suffered from soul sickness. (Alison refers to broken souls.) I know that addiction isolates. Back in 1987, I found myself imprisoned (and isolated) within the glass walls of a cocaine vial. Love healed my soul; and as you will see, my story is not unique. My first connection came from the love of my brothers and sisters in recovery, then love from my family, and finally love from a power greater than myself. Then again, I may have that completely backward.

Addiction isolates. Recovery connects.

Recovery Allies prompts some deep questions. I appreciate that so much. As a recovery coach, I always strive for the best question to ask in any given situation. Notice I did not say to provide the best answer. Some of the questions I find myself asking now are:

Where will people connect in the future?

How can we foster more healing connection in our communities?

How can we better love our neighbors?

Recovery Allies has the potential to open hearts and minds to new possibilities. Take what you need, and leave the rest. Then I urge you to move forward and do your part to create a community around you that is recovery friendly.

Phillip Valentine, Recovery Coach Professional
Executive Director
Connecticut Community for Addiction
Recovery (CCAR)

PREFACE

At a Maine Harm Reduction Conference a few years ago, a burly, athletic man in his thirties who was finishing his degree in social work talked about stigma and how the language we choose really matters. "When you call me an addict, you take away everything that is lovely about me," he said. Four months later, he died from a drug overdose. His friends think he was too ashamed of his return to heroin use to ask for help. He left behind a son, girlfriend, mother, siblings, and scores of people he had helped as a case worker at a homeless shelter during his four years of sobriety.

It doesn't have to be this way. There are far more recovery success stories than stories of unrelenting addiction and death. Recovery is possible and even probable, and we all have a part in creating conditions where healing and hope can flourish. In my work as a recovery advocate, I've learned the many ways that we as community members, together with people in recovery, can harness our resources to build a community response to addiction that makes our neighborhoods, towns, and cities healthy places for people to begin and sustain new lives in recovery.

I learned a lot about recovery a few years ago from a team of college students in Portland, Maine. Bryn, Andrew, Matt, and Alex worked with me on a project to increase treatment and recovery services for youth across the state. One strategy was to go around the state and hold community meetings to talk about addiction and recovery. Together with Anna Black, the project director, we traveled around Maine, and they told their recovery stories in school gyms and cafeterias, performance halls, and conference rooms. After they spoke, people had a chance to ask questions, and invariably someone would come up to me after the meeting and ask, "What can I do to help?" This book answers that question.

Getting to know "the crew" came at a time when my own children had finished college and were living out of state. I missed my kids, and these students filled a massive gap in my heart. When I wasn't around, they called me "Mama Webb." We had a lot of laughs over the two-year project, and they taught me what it's like to be a young adult in recovery today. They also taught me a lot about being a recovery ally. I was ready for a change in my career direction, and working on recovery support felt right. I never dreamed it would take me along a path of learning, joy, and deep sorrow. I learned more about my family and my attitudes toward addiction and about nonjudgmental empathy and how hard that is to give sometimes. Along the way, my passion for social justice expanded. This book is part of that journey.

Even though addiction runs in my family, the term "recovery" was new to me. I'm a granddaughter, niece, aunt, sibling, and cousin of people with addiction, some in recovery, and I had never heard the word used in my family. If we talked about substance use at all, it was in whispers and with words like "drunk" and "junkie," but most of the time, we just didn't talk about it. The specter of men who didn't enter recovery and died because of their addiction was always slinking around the dark corners of family life. I didn't learn about empathy and compassion for people with a substance use disorder; I learned how to judge their moral failings.

Since 2015, I have conducted several focus groups and interviewed more than fifty people of all ages in—and at all stages of—recovery. *Recovery Allies* uses the results of those focus groups and interviews to describe recovery as people live it. In all of these discussions, we spent a limited time talking about drug and alcohol use, which is provided here only for context, and most of our time talking about recovery. Participants told me their stories about rebuilding their lives, not just on the outside, but inside where fears, anxiety, anger, and broken souls reside. They worked to repair relationships and own up to their conduct and behavior that wasn't consistent with their own values or community values. They found a way to manage the shame. For this book, I took what people told me, what they chose to share, and organized it by themes. These stories put power into the hands of people in recovery and show their family members and the larger community what they need to stay well. I hope the reader doesn't see this as appropriating their stories for a professional end, but instead as I intend it—to get other people to understand their lives and engage in creating recovery-friendly communities.

Consistent threads turned up in these conversations and are woven throughout this book. They are:

Stigma is a powerful force.

Substance use disorder is one of the most stigmatized conditions across the globe, and the stigma surrounding it keeps people in active addiction from seeking help. It keeps family members silent in their pain and grief. It lives on in recovery in the forms of low expectations for success, snide comments about the past, and outright discrimination in housing and employment.

Peers are more important than professionals.

Nearly everyone I spoke with acknowledged the help of counselors and health care providers in their treatment and transition into recovery, but they were adamant that they couldn't have sustained their recovery without compassion and encouragement from peers who have "been there," who "get it" when the going gets tough, and who know when to celebrate small changes that add up to a full life in recovery.

It's about the conditions that lead to addiction, not the drug.

In the current environment of opioid overdose deaths, the media and people in positions of power have focused attention on prescription painkillers, heroin, and fentanyl. This focus misses the point: addiction is killing Americans. One of the people I interviewed was clear on this subject. "We need to start focusing on the real problems: poverty and mental illness instead of the drug. People say, 'Heroin is ruining our community,' when really, there was a problem well before heroin came around."

The voice of families is powerful.

Parents who have lost children to drug overdose have braved stigma, grief, and disappointment to speak up in their communities and lobby policy makers at state and federal levels to prevent more deaths. Now, parents whose children are in recovery and other family members join them to talk about what they need to support the people they love. Advocacy organizations have brought families together to tell their stories, and decision makers have started to listen to them.

Allies are important.

Every national advocate I spoke with said, "We can't do it without allies." Advocates need people with a heart for recovery who will use their skills, resources, and positions to improve the lives of people in recovery.

Recovery is political.

People in recovery come from across the political spectrum, and supporting recovery isn't an issue that the political right or the political left can own. While progressives argue for an end to the drug war and conservatives want more enforcement of existing drug laws, we have to focus on common ground. Community-based recovery support services and help for families who are struggling are issues we can all get behind.

We can't expect people in power to change the system.

We have to make them do it. We have to insist on a place at the decision-making table for people in recovery and their allies. We know what people in the community need to support sustained recovery, and we must advocate for it. We need to use what we know from research to force funding more effective treatment and recovery support services.

Communities have abundant capacity to act.

Communities can be more responsive to local needs than state and federal agencies, private insurance companies, and private foundations that fund most substance use disorder treatment and recovery support services. While local assets—like personal networks, recovery champions, coalitions, businesses, and the faith community—vary considerably across the country, every community has them. It's up to community members to find a way to tap into their unique assets to support recovery in a way that makes sense locally, without waiting for governmental agencies and large private entities to act.

Communities benefit from being recovery friendly.

Supporting people in recovery isn't a one-way street. Research shows that recovery-friendly communities benefit from greater volunteerism and community participation, and a loyal workforce.

○ ○ ○

Recovery Allies touches on essential actions to build recovery-friendly communities today. It's not exhaustive. I haven't addressed recovery among immigrants or communities of color in depth. I believe someone from those communities should do that work. I haven't addressed process addictions like gambling. I haven't done justice to the relationship between addiction and mental health, addiction and incarceration, addiction and trauma, or the incredibly damaging impact of addiction on young children in families where parents and other adults use substances. These were in the background of my interviews, but we focused on recovery *today*. Wherever possible, I have discussed social justice issues as they relate to recovery. The topic deserves full-fledged research and advocacy for marginalized people and others who have limited opportunities to get well.

In this book, I argue for a public health approach to recovery to create recovery-friendly communities. Many people have called for a public health response to "our opioid crisis" and, more generally, to addiction. Our federal and state governments haven't stepped up with an effective public health response. For better or worse, that creates opportunities for people in communities to do the job. We know that when we give people hope, help, love, and quality treatment within their window of willingness, they recover. I think our job is to understand what recovery means to our loved ones, friends, and neighbors and create a supportive environment so they can stay the course on their journey.

I thank everyone who talked with me about their experiences. The conversations were intimate, joyful, and so meaningful. I learned that when you enter the recovery community, you're welcomed into a big family full of love, support, and heated disagreements, just like any family. There's no better way to understand the recovery journey for people who aren't in recovery than to ask, and then listen. When we do, we create an opportunity to see the world through someone else's eyes. We're all works in progress, figuring out our place in the world. Appreciating our differences goes a long way toward coming together as a community and learning how to take care of each other.

When I asked, "What can community members do?" the people I interviewed all said, "Get educated." This book will help do just that. They also said, "Get involved," "Be an ally," and "Help reduce stigma."

Let's get to work.

Section 1
Recovery Basics

INTRODUCTION TO
THE RECOVERY ECOSYSTEM

RECOVERY ALLIES IS a book of uncomfortable truths. On one hand, we'll see that individuals recover from addiction through their hard work and by figuring out how to live without the substances that created chaos in their lives. On the other hand, we'll see that they *don't* recover on their own; their recovery is a meaningful and growing relationship with their friends, families, and the community where they live. We'll see that *most* people with substance use disorders resolve their problems, and that recovery is not only possible, it's *probable.* Yet, people who recover are not distributed equally in all communities, and circumstances like poverty, unemployment, discrimination, trauma, and social isolation create conditions that make healing from addiction less likely. Opioid overdose deaths created a crisis that forced policy makers to address opioid addiction in our communities and increase access to treatment and prevent deaths. But their focus on opioids pulled attention away from the fact that our problem isn't just an opioid crisis; it's an *addiction* crisis.

All of these are true at the same time.

In the United States, we treat addiction as an acute medical problem to be solved with bouts of intense treatment followed by periods of abstinence, relapse, and then treatment again. This unfortunate "acute care/relapse" pattern is like prescribing a rescue inhaler as a permanent solution for a child who experiences a serious asthma attack. The immediate problem may go away, but the inhaler doesn't address the underlying causes of the attack, which could be from living in substandard housing or an urban area with high pollution levels or seasonal allergies—or some combination.

Public health research shows that socioeconomic factors like education, income, race, and ethnicity are more critical influences affecting health than clinical interventions. One study found that socioeconomic factors account for nearly half of health outcomes, while clinical care accounts for less than one-fifth.[1] So, while anyone can get asthma, including people from healthy living environments, the condition isn't distributed equally across all populations. Stress, violence, and socioeconomic status of individuals, households, and communities have given rise to environments that create risks for asthma and a cluster of other chronic diseases.[2] Just as sending an asthma patient back into an unhealthy environment with an inhaler as treatment doesn't address asthma as a chronic illness, sending a person from substance use treatment back into a community that still has the circumstances that created depression, anxiety, and trauma with an individualized recovery plan doesn't do much to address addiction as a chronic condition.

In public health, we see individuals as part of a complex web of individual characteristics, family relationships, social networks, cultural norms, and economic factors that create the social determinants of health. In the context of recovery, we think about the "recovery ecosystem" (aspects of community life that can promote recovery) and "recovery capital" (the sum total of the assets an individual brings to recovery) as those social determinants.[3] And we all live in this recovery ecosystem. We can create a recovery desert, hostile to people in recovery, or a recovery-friendly community. We can make conditions better for people seeking or in recovery, or we can make them worse. We can be supportive of recovery or not.

Recovery Allies is about community members getting involved in the lives of people in recovery and their families to make communities healthier for everybody. It's about mobilizing community capital and making it accessible to people who don't have connections or resources to get the support and assistance they need for their recovery. In the same way that we want our communities to support the needs of the elderly, or high school students, or young parents, or any other group, we want them to support people in

recovery. When we step back as community members and let treatment providers, social workers, drug court lawyers, judges, and health care and other
professionals do all the heavy lifting, we shouldn't be surprised when the
results fall short. Their collective work, while needed and so beneficial, isn't
sufficient to address addiction in our communities.

Healthy relationships with and support from the broader community,
recovery support services, opportunities for work, education, volunteering,
and being part of a spiritual group can make a tremendous difference to
individuals in recovery. When we contribute to these aspects of recovery, we
create recovery-friendly communities, and we become essential partners in
the recovery of the people we love.

A Public Health Approach to Recovery

Public health is a social and political undertaking. It's what we, as a society,
do collectively to ensure the conditions in which people can be healthy.[4]
*A recovery-friendly community is a social and political undertaking that we engage
in collectively to promote the conditions in which people in and seeking recovery can
be healthy.*

In 2016, the Office of the Surgeon General published a landmark report:
*Facing Addiction in America: The Surgeon General's Report on Alcohol, Drugs,
and Health.* The authors of this document—the first-ever Surgeon General's report on the topic and free to the public—created a one-stop shop for
questions, answers, and source materials. *Facing Addiction* acknowledges that,
despite decades of dealing with substance use through the criminal justice
system, "substance misuse remains a public health crisis that continues to
rob the United States of its most valuable asset: its people." The report calls
for a public health systems approach to our substance misuse problem. This
means that community leaders work together to "mobilize the capacities of
health care organizations, social service organizations, educational systems,
community-based organizations, government health agencies, religious institutions, law enforcement, local businesses, researchers, and other public, private, and voluntary entities." Together, this team (1) uses data to define the
problem of substance misuse; (2) identifies factors that increase or decrease
the risk for substance misuse; (3) works across the public and private sectors

to develop interventions (programs, services, or policies) to address the social, environmental, or economic determinants of substance misuse; (4) supports effective prevention and treatment interventions and recovery supports; and (5) monitors the impact of these interventions.[5]

Recovery Allies seconds that determination and goes further by calling for a community-based public health approach to recovery. Here, the team of community leaders will center its focus on recovery and (1) use data to define the problem of poor recovery outcomes; (2) identify factors that increase or decrease the chances for successful recovery outcomes; (3) work across the public and private sectors to develop interventions (programs, services, or policies) to address the social, environmental, or economic determinants of recovery; (4) support effective recovery support services and other interventions; and (5) monitor the impact of these interventions. The book aims to educate readers, using personal stories of recovery, providing data and research, and offering examples of community interventions to demonstrate how community members can be part of this process.

Professionals on the front lines of the opioid crisis have called for a public health approach to the opioid problem. Law enforcement officers have declared that "we can't arrest our way out of this problem," referring to the opioid crisis and sheer number of people with drug-related charges and convictions in the criminal justice system, and have appealed for prevention services and access to treatment.[6] Media attention to the rapid rise in drug overdose deaths in the 2010s grabbed the attention of policy makers, who followed researchers' recommendations for a multipronged approach that includes changing prescribing practices, disposing of prescription drugs, making treatment available, and making naloxone (a medication that may reverse opioid overdoses) widely available.[7] So far, these calls for action have had mixed and disappointing results.[8]

This focus on opioids and overdose deaths is essential, of course, but it's partial and misleading. It ignores the fact that overdose deaths have been increasing exponentially since 1979, well before the large increase in opioid prescribing.[9] It also ignores the fact that most people who receive an opioid prescription from a doctor don't develop an opioid use disorder.[10] It downplays the more than 72,000 deaths caused by the most-used substance—alcohol—each year in the United States[11] and has drawn attention away from the larger truth that we don't just have an opioid crisis; we have an *addiction* crisis. To put it another way, if we were to reduce opioid overdose deaths to zero, could we really say that we had succeeded when addiction continues unabated? It may seem obvious, but bears saying: Reducing overdose deaths is a starting point and not a goal in itself. Reversing overdoses and then sending people with opioid use disorder back into the same circumstances that created the problem in the first place is madness. We do a disservice to people with addictions and their families when *in addition to preventing overdoses* we don't focus on supporting their recoveries. Would we declare success if we visited the scene of a car accident and applied tourniquets to stop the bleeding of the injured, but left them at the scene?

Single-minded attention to opioid overdose deaths focuses on end-stage substance use disorder. It centers the problem on the substance—its deadly qualities, who prescribes it, who sells it, who uses it—rather than on the *reason* people use it. In public health, we focus less on the drug and more on the context, the environment, and the mental health of people who use drugs.[12] This context includes the cluster of psychological, medical, family, and social problems, with trauma, mental health, and a lack of resources at the top of the list. These are often called the "root causes" of addiction.[13] When we understand why people use drugs and alcohol and work on supporting their recoveries, we stand a better chance of solving our overarching addiction crisis.

The Role of Allies

Allies play a crucial role in addressing addiction in our communities. Although there's no single definition, a recovery ally generally is a passionate supporter of and advocate for individuals in recovery and for the recovery community as a whole. There are many ways to be one. As allies, we use our assets, skills, resources, and connections to work side by side with the recovery community to build recovery-friendly communities. We learn about addiction and recovery, and we keep up with new trends in recovery support services. We invite people in recovery into our places of work and worship. We help create a healthy environment for people at all stages of recovery. We show up at public events and speak in support of people in recovery. We speak out against stigma.

As allies, we create safe spaces to talk about addiction and recovery. When we understand why people struggle in recovery, we can look at ways to support them on their journeys. We do this by asking them, with genuine compassion and curiosity, how they heal best, what they need, and how we can support them, and then we listen to their answers. As allies, we may know the stories of one or two close friends or family members, but we need to go further and find out about other pathways. Then we can work to provide evidence-based recovery support services and opportunities for individuals to increase their recovery capital. Finally, we can put our efforts into changing the community environment—our policies, practices, and social and cultural norms—that created the conditions for substance use in the first place. When we do all of this, we extend our focus from the individual's recovery to building the social, economic, and cultural conditions that foster health and well-being.

About This Book

Recovery Allies embraces the addiction field's paradigm shift from focusing on the pathology of addiction to supporting long-term recovery. This shift urges us to explore the positive experiences of people in recovery to understand how they resolve addiction in real life.[14] *Recovery Allies* is in solidarity with US Surgeon General Vivek Murthy's *Together: The Healing Power of Human Connection in a Sometimes Lonely World,* a book that emphasizes the importance of authentic and caring human relationships, not just for those with addictions and in recovery, but for all of us.[15] *Recovery Allies* takes as truth journalist Johann Hari's now-famous statement: "The opposite of addiction isn't sobriety. It's connection."[16]

Recovery Allies is informed by science, research, and the narratives of people in recovery. Like other works in public health advocacy, it draws on findings from many fields of research and practice, including neuroscience, sociology, psychology, and trauma. The nature of public health is to take a holistic view. In the case of people in recovery, we're not just concerned about whether they use substances or the status of their neurochemistry. We're interested in all aspects of their lives and creating healthy conditions for them to live successfully in a welcoming community.

Central to this approach is cultural humility, which calls on all of us to reflect on our biases about people who use drugs and people in recovery.

Addiction disproportionately impacts people who are homeless, people who were incarcerated, and communities of color. Cultural humility implores us to appreciate others' points of view, interrogate our own positions on issues like drug policy and harm reduction, and consider how the root causes of addiction impact people's lives.

No single book can describe the full range of recovery experiences. I've sought as much variety in my interviews as possible, and the voices in this book reveal diverse recovery experiences. Every person's recovery is different, and one of this book's goals is to honor those differences.

I interviewed more than fifty people for this book—researchers, community leaders, allies, advocates, and most importantly, people in recovery and the friends and family members who love them. They all talked with me about their experiences, successes, frustrations, and hopes for the future. I asked each person what communities can do to support recovery, and their answers form the core of this book.

These hours of conversations focused on recovery; there were few war stories about what happened in active addiction. The dreary and sometimes disastrous periods in active use are a small part of the narrative here. I recognize the ravages that addiction creates for individuals, families, and communities and that relapses can be terrifying and deadly. I acknowledge that some people with addictions will never choose recovery and that some who choose it aren't able to sustain it. There are many, many books about addiction and the damage it causes. I've taken another path: writing about recovery and the joys it can bring, with details about periods of active addiction included only for context.

Recovery Allies is about people with addiction who typically have less recovery capital—fewer assets to support their recovery—than people with less severe problems. Many of the community actions and recovery support services described in this book will be of most help to people who are in recovery from addiction. Other community actions, like using nonstigmatizing language and creating safe spaces to talk about drug and alcohol problems, may benefit people who have resolved less severe issues.

Communities are different. Even in the age of the internet, drug use and recovery pathways vary by region and community, and generalities miss those variations. In some communities, religion is an important part of recovery and in others it's not. Some communities have a high rate of opioid use disorder, and others don't. No matter what region or community, there are never enough resources to solve community problems. That's just part of the challenge of making changes so our communities are recovery friendly. We have to start where we are—where else could we start?—and create the best environment for people in recovery and the people who love them that we can, given the limitations we face. Parts of *Recovery Allies* will resonate with some readers and not others. The best way to use this book is to follow the advice often heard in Alcoholics Anonymous meetings: "Take what's helpful and leave the rest."

Recovery Allies is divided into eight sections:

1. Recovery Basics

Recovery from what? *Recovery Allies* is about people with the most severe substance use disorder: addiction. The compulsion to use—not being able to stop even in the face of disastrous consequences—is the hallmark of addiction and separates people with addiction from everyone else who uses substances. This section provides essential background information on defining addiction, which isn't as straightforward as it might seem. Terms we use in an environment of changing norms about language are defined, and we cover how people in recovery define it. We'll see that not everyone thinks about it the same way and that there are many facets to recovery. This section also describes recovery research to date and directions for future investigations.

2. Recovery-Friendly Communities

Section 2 discusses the importance of building recovery capital and recovery-friendly communities. Recovery capital is the sum of the assets people bring to their recovery and includes self-esteem, social relationships, financial means, education, employment, and resources available in the broader community that support recovery, like policies for safe housing and drug sentencing laws. This section explores how allies can help create and expand recovery capital. It also includes examples of public health strategies that some communities have taken, using recovery as an organizing principle, to increase recovery capital and build recovery-friendly communities.

3. The Recovery Journey

Each chapter of the third section informs the reader about a recovery topic based on experiences of people in recovery and scientific research:

Pathways of Recovery

"Multiple pathways of recovery" is a phrase that people in the recovery field use to talk about the many ways people sustain their recovery. This chapter uses narratives of people in recovery and insights from recovery research to illustrate some of those pathways. Not everyone follows well-worn paths; some people forge their own way forward. Saying "you're in recovery when you say you are" gets at the heart of recovery as a self-defined path to wellness.

Alcoholics Anonymous and 12-Step Programs

Alcoholics Anonymous (AA) is the principal foundation for recovery in America and may be the most well-known pathway. This part of section 3 describes what it's like to participate in AA and summarizes research confirming that AA is an effective tool to help people with alcohol use disorder.

Recovery and Stigma

Substance use disorders are one of the most stigmatized human conditions, and that stigma continues to be borne by those who are healing from addiction. Stigma and discrimination create barriers to health care, housing, and other basic needs essential in early recovery. In addition, having a record of arrests and convictions can be a barrier to education and meaningful work. This part of section 3 describes shame, social stigma, discrimination, and the changes that allies can make to reduce stigma.

Harm Reduction

Harm reduction has expanded outside traditional boundaries of overdose prevention and the provision of clean needles and other supplies to people who inject drugs while they are using. This part of section 3 describes new approaches to harm reduction, including controversial subjects like safe injection sites, the call for decriminalization of drugs, and the radical notion that "harm reduction is love."

Recovery, Trauma, and Mental Illness

People with drug and alcohol addictions often have a history of trauma or mental illness. For some of them, life in recovery is difficult, especially when the long-term effects of previously prescribed psychiatric medications are present. While their narratives are hopeful, they're not always the recovery stories they would have wished for.

4. The Pillars of Recovery: Health

The four pillars of recovery identified as essential by the federal Substance Abuse and Mental Health Services Administration—Health, Home, Purpose, and Community—form the basis for this and the following three sections.

People in recovery have health conditions and concerns that result from years of using substances. Section 4 discusses health and wellness in people in recovery. It also touches on personal experiences of some of the many people who find healing power in religion and spirituality during recovery. And it briefly explains why medications like methadone and buprenorphine—two of the most common prescription medications for opioid addiction—are the foundation for recovery for many people. (Buprenorphine is available in several formulations. Suboxone is the trade name for one of those, and the word is used commonly in the recovery community to refer to any formulation of buprenorphine.)

5. The Pillars of Recovery: Home

Safe housing for people in early recovery often means an alcohol- and drug-free living environment where they can create new and healthy relationships and behaviors. Section 5 explores how to find quality recovery housing—and some of the pitfalls—and what communities can do to support recovery residences. It also addresses special housing needs for women in recovery and barriers people with felony convictions have in accessing housing in the rental market.

6. The Pillars of Recovery: Purpose

Living in recovery means finding meaning in your life, finding your "why." Section 6 describes how work and volunteering are ways people in recovery contribute to their community, build recovery capital, reintegrate, and find meaning and dignity. It also gets into how education is important for building self-esteem, fostering intellectual growth, and creating a career path. Recovery centers on university and college campuses support students in an environment of rampant drug and alcohol use. And a note on fulfillment describes the joy that often comes after several years of sustained recovery.

7. The Pillars of Recovery: Community

Research shows that peer support is an essential aspect of recovery; many people in long-term recovery say their peers were more important to their recovery than any professional help was. This section describes formal and informal peer relationships, recovery community centers, and other avenues for peer support.

8. Recovery Advocacy

The final section describes how recovery is a personal journey that is most successful in communities willing to step up to the challenges of being recovery friendly. National, state, and local organizations are part of the New Recovery Advocacy Movement to change policies to support recovery. Recovery isn't an issue for the political right or the political left; it's an issue that impacts people across the political spectrum. Allies can be part of changing policies to create recovery-friendly communities.

Most chapters of *Recovery Allies* end with a list of concrete actions readers can take to create recovery-friendly communities. In developing these action steps, I have tried to be faithful to my training as a recovery coach—to treat people in recovery as a resource in their own recovery, not like a vessel that needs to be filled with someone else's help. Readers in a hurry to *do something* can cut to the chase and go directly to this last part of each chapter. Recommended actions stem from core public health strategies, recovery research, and suggestions from the people I interviewed. Generally, they fall into four categories worth emphasizing:

1. Learn about recovery.
2. Help reduce stigma.
3. Get involved by being a recovery ally.
4. Identify your own strengths and use them to create a recovery-friendly community.

2

RECOVERY FROM WHAT?

THIS BOOK IS about recovery from drug and alcohol addiction. Terminology can be confusing. Fuzzy thinking, new research, changing definitions, and our general overuse of the word "addiction" to mean an attachment to just about anything we love all contribute to misunderstandings of what addiction actually means.

Scientists and health care providers claim addiction is a chronic, relapsing medical condition. Social scientists are more interested in the social causes of drug use, like poverty, racism, and lack of access to substance use treatment and mental health counseling. Some people of faith focus on a broken relationship with God. People in recovery talk about a miserable life while they were using. We're like the blind men trying to figure out what the elephant is. The man who touched its leg thought the elephant was a pillar. The man who touched the ears thought the elephant was a big fan. In reality, no one could see the whole elephant. We claim to know the truth based on our limited experience and knowledge while ignoring other people's experiences and expertise when all may be true at the same time.

Trying to figure out what addiction is often leads to simplistic or reductionist thinking. We hear people say, "It's all in the genes," or "It's a brain disease," or "They have an addictive personality," or "They're self-medicating." In the end, we're all looking at a complex aspect of the human condition, trying to understand why some people continue to use alcohol or drugs even when the consequences are dire. Unraveling this mystery has riveted researchers, writers, and people of faith and plagued family members and communities for ages. Current thinking points to some combination of changes in the brain due to drug use, genetic vulnerabilities, socioeconomic factors, underlying mental and physical health of individuals, and the social context of drug use. This section briefly discusses the dominant understandings of addiction and the implications for communities creating conditions for recovery.

A NOTE ON LANGUAGE

In general, this book uses terminology that people in recovery use when speaking in public about addiction. (Their language behind closed doors, with other people in recovery, may be different.) Often, they refer to times when they were using drugs or alcohol as "being in active addiction" or "using," rather than substance abuse or misuse. They refer to "return to use" or "recurrence of symptoms" or "slip" when they are back in active addiction. Some people use the term "relapse," although some in the recovery community consider it stigmatizing. (A "slip" usually means a short return to use followed by seeking help and returning to recovery quickly. "Relapse" usually means a longer return to use, with little interest in a life in recovery.) They say "addiction" to refer to severe substance use disorder, and this book will do the same. *Recovery Allies* will refer to "having a drug problem" or "having a problem with alcohol" for mild or moderate substance use disorders.

The current thinking is that person-first language—saying "a person with a substance use disorder" or "a person with a problem with alcohol"—delivers a less harmful message than saying alcoholic, addict, or substance abuser. Here are some other considerations on use of language.[1]

- **Substance use**—a general, nonstigmatizing, nonjudgmental, non-clinical term

- **Substance abuse**—an older term still in use but felt to be stigmatizing by some in the recovery community

- **Substance misuse**—a nonclinical term that implies a correct and incorrect way to use substances

- **Problematic or chaotic substance use**—a nonclinical term, used by some harm reductionists

- **Substance use disorder**—a clinical/medical term that many people use to describe a severe form of the disease

- **Addiction/alcoholism**—nonclinical terms that usually refer to people with the most severe problem

---

What Is Addiction?

For everyone, substance use occurs along a continuum—from abstinence to experimentation, occasional use, regular use, heavy use, problematic use, and chaotic use. Addiction happens when drug or alcohol use becomes uncontrollable and creates chaos in a person's life.

The American Psychiatric Association's *Diagnostic and Statistical Manual of Mental Disorders,* 5th edition *(DSM-5)* provides the current diagnostic criteria for substance use disorder (SUD), the clinical term now in use, listed below. It reflects the scientific consensus of changing understandings of mental health and substance use conditions. A person with fewer than two symptoms has no SUD. A person with two or three symptoms has a mild disorder. A person with four or five symptoms has a moderate disorder, and a person with six or more has a severe disorder (informally referred to as addiction).[2, 3]

1. Using in larger amounts or for longer than intended

2. Wanting to cut down or stop using, but not managing to

3. Spending a lot of time to get, use, or recover from use

4. Craving

5. Inability to manage commitments due to use

6. Continuing to use, even when it causes problems in relationships

7. Giving up important activities because of use

8. Continuing to use, even when it puts you in danger

9. Continuing to use, even when physical or psychological problems may be made worse by use

10. Increasing tolerance

11. Withdrawal symptoms

Severe SUD (addiction) results from prolonged, repeated use of substances at high doses or high frequencies. People with a less severe problem typically have no family history of substance use, a later onset of use (usually after the teenage years), fewer and less severe issues associated with use, fewer medical and mental health comorbidities, and more family and social supports.[4] This doesn't mean their substance use hasn't caused problems. People without a diagnosis of severe SUD can and do use substances that create problems for themselves and their communities. For example, occasional binge drinking may result in car crashes, domestic violence, or other social issues but doesn't rise to the level of a severe SUD.[5]

It's important to note that these symptoms are for drug or alcohol problems only. Untangling problems with substances from mental health issues like depression or anxiety is complicated. Some people just have a problem with substances. Still, most people who have a diagnosable severe SUD have some co-occurring mental health condition or have experienced trauma in their lives. Sometimes, the extent of the mental health issue isn't fully understood until substances are taken out of the equation.

These diagnostic criteria have enormous real-world consequences. In theory, a proper diagnosis leads to appropriate treatment, but it doesn't always happen that way. The US Surgeon General estimates that only 10 percent of people with SUD of any severity get treatment in any one year, and only 25 percent of people with SUD receive specialized treatment in their lifetime.[6] *The vast majority of people with substance use disorder don't receive proper care for their condition, which means tens of thousands of people go without help every year.*

Diagnostic criteria are also critical because they form the basis for reimbursement of addiction treatment in public insurance programs (Medicaid and Medicare, for example) and the private insurance industry. As health care providers like hospitals roll out recovery support services for patients, a substance use disorder diagnosis may be part of the debate about reimbursement rates for recovery coaches and other forms of recovery support services.

Models of Addiction

The **brain disease model** of addiction is currently the leading explanation for why some people develop problems using drugs or alcohol.[7] We can sum up the model like this: Addiction impacts parts of the brain that control planning and organization, decision making, memory, self-awareness, impulse control, emotional regulation, and reward (pleasure) seeking. A person with a brain impaired by addiction has a compromised ability to stop using drugs even when drug use consequences are disastrous. While proponents of the disease model acknowledge that addiction starts with a choice to use drugs and that other influences including genetics and childhood experiences like neglect and sexual abuse play a role, brain impairment is at the center of understanding.

Addiction is a condition that changes the way the brain works. After drug use ceases, the brain heals and recovers over time from the toxic effects of drugs and alcohol and may return to normal functioning. Research on how this healing happens is in its infancy, so we don't know much about it.[8] In the meantime, treating addiction is like treating diabetes—recognizing there is no cure and focusing on chronic disease management, including reducing symptoms (which include using drugs or alcohol); improving physical, mental, and social functioning; and preventing relapse. Recovery happens with appropriate medications that help the brain heal; behavioral therapies such as individual, group, and family counseling; and recovery support services.

The National Institute on Drug Abuse (NIDA), the largest funder of addiction research in the United States, promotes and supports the brain disease model. NIDA's definition of addiction is: "a chronic, relapsing disorder characterized by compulsive drug seeking, continued use despite harmful consequences, and long-lasting changes in the brain. It is considered both a complex brain disorder and a mental illness. Addiction is the most severe form of a full spectrum of substance use disorders, and is a medical illness caused by repeated misuse of a substance or substances."[9]

The brain disease model aligns with an older and less scientific view of "the disease of addiction" espoused by Alcoholics Anonymous (AA) since the 1930s—alcoholism as a **"spiritual malady"** as well as a physical illness. The inability to control drinking is a symptom of this spiritual disease. AA's 12 steps form a powerful spiritual path to sobriety, recovery, and being "spiritually fit." Many people in the recovery community, including nonreligious people and those outside the 12-step community, see the spiritual aspect as paramount: addiction happens when "you have a hole in your heart that you try to fill with drugs or alcohol."

Researchers and practitioners of the **biopsychosocial model** consider the focus on brain chemistry too narrow and reductionist. They broaden the explanation of why some people develop drug and alcohol problems to include biological factors (especially having a family history of addiction), psychological factors (experiencing trauma, especially in childhood), psychiatric factors (underlying mental health conditions), and social factors (such as being in a social environment that promotes drug use). The combination of biopsychosocial factors determines who ends up with addiction. [10, 11, 12, 13]

The American Society of Addiction Medicine (ASAM), the national organization that represents physicians, clinicians, and other professionals in the field of addiction medicine, incorporated both the brain disease and the biopsychosocial models in its definition of addiction in 2019. ASAM now defines addiction as: "a treatable, chronic medical disease involving complex interactions among brain circuits, genetics, the environment, and an individual's life experiences. People with addiction use substances or engage in behaviors that become compulsive and often continue despite harmful consequences. Prevention efforts and treatment approaches for addiction are generally as successful as those for other chronic diseases."[14]

Many researchers think that the brain disease model fails to adequately take into account broad social factors leading to addiction.[15] Bruce Alexander, a psychologist known for his research on addiction, has advanced the **dislocation theory of addiction,** which identifies addiction as an adaptive response to social structures in a globalized world that "dislocate individuals" from their sense of meaning, purpose, and value.[16] For Gabor Maté, an addiction physician in Vancouver, Canada, the question isn't "Why the addiction?" but "Why the pain?" Why do people seek to dull emotional pain with substances and compulsive behaviors?[17] Drugs meet the needs that people have for pain relief and connection that post-capitalistic society can't meet. Maté and others challenge the view that addiction is primarily a biological, inherited condition treatable with appropriate clinical interventions. There may be a genetic predisposition, but not predetermination. They suggest a paradigm shift. A different, broader view is that our social system creates trauma and alienation, and seeking to "fix individuals" through treatment is no solution. Instead, we need to change the social system to address basic human needs for connection and safety to avoid human suffering in the first place.[18, 19]

For Native Americans and other communities that have experienced massive losses of lives and culture and Black American communities with a history of slavery and racism, addiction is one of the many results of **intergenerational trauma.** Healing from addiction isn't just the individual's responsibility; individuals, families, and communities are healing together from this unresolved historical trauma and historical grief in ways that incorporate culture, a return to tradition, and spiritual empowerment.[20]

The **moral model of addiction** holds that addiction is a choice, and people with addictions are morally flawed. While the scientific community doesn't embrace this view, it is maintained to some degree in the general population and contributes significantly to addiction stigma. In some religions, addiction is a sin. For some Christians, we're all sinners—addiction is one among many sins—and we're all in need of redemption.[21] In some Christian communities, addiction and its consequences are considered a faith test that disappears through deepened faith and spiritual practice.[22]

What Can Allies Do?

If we're going to create a recovery-friendly community, we need to understand the different ways of thinking and beliefs about addiction. Whether we agree with other people's views about the causes of addiction or not, understanding that there are different ways of thinking means there are various resources in our community like doctors, counselors, and faith groups to support various aspects of recovery. Once we know about these options, we'll feel more comfortable talking about solutions.

For Everyone

- Before jumping into action, take a moment and consider how you think about addiction. Do you think there's something wrong with a person who can't stop using drugs or alcohol? Do you think their brains are just wired wrong? Do you believe they're morally corrupt? Or do you think they're sick and need help?

- Think about your own drug and alcohol use. Do you drink or use drugs to relieve stress or to remove inhibitions in social situations? Has your use ever gotten out of control? Have you ever done dangerous or foolish things while you were under the influence? Have you ever been worried about how much you use? Do you think it's immoral to drink or use drugs?

- Consider your own experiences with people who have a substance use disorder. Stepping back from your own emotions that you have toward someone with a severe drug or alcohol problem— anger, disgust, resentment, sadness—can help you think more clearly about their addiction and the consequences in their life.

- Learn about substance use disorder. Understanding that it's a diagnosable condition that can be mild, moderate, or severe means that not everyone who drinks a lot or smokes cannabis has an addiction. It also means that different treatments are appropriate for different people.

- Learn about the disease model. Understanding that addiction is a chronic, relapsing disorder characterized by long-lasting changes in the brain may help us see why some people "just can't quit." It can help us find just a bit more compassion when their drug use continues in the face of obvious consequences like broken relationships, arrests, and lost jobs.

- Learn about the biopsychosocial model, which can help us see just how complex addiction is. Growing up in a household or neighborhood where drug use and violence were the norms, living in poverty, or living without meaning and purpose can contribute to initiating and continuing drug use. Current circumstances like living in isolation or a community experiencing intergenerational trauma make it hard to find a path out of addiction.

- Learn about the moral model of addiction. Understanding that some people see addiction as a moral weakness or spiritual test helps us know the shame that people in active addiction feel and the potentially redeeming balm that religion and spirituality can offer.

3

RECOVERY DEFINED

I ASKED EACH of the people I interviewed for this book, "What does recovery mean to you?" Here are some of their answers:

> "I think of hope. Recovery equals the power of possibility. You go from the addiction world where you're told, 'You can't, and you won't.' Then you get to the treatment world where you are told, 'You can't, you're not, you can't be.' But once you are in recovery, you're told, 'You can, and you will!'"
>
> —THIRTY-FIVE-YEAR-OLD MAN

> "To the extent that any of us can determine where our life is going—the human experience—that is recovery. It's the human experience."
>
> —FIFTY-YEAR-OLD MAN

> "I think of an individualized process of trying to work towards a goal of happiness and comfortability in life. The point I try to convey is that while people try to force their ideas of recovery on you, ultimately, each individual is to decide what their recovery looks like as long as they are comfortable in their own skin and exhibiting a relatively acceptable amount of psychosocial functioning."
>
> —THIRTY-FIVE-YEAR-OLD MAN

"When I see a person in recovery who has what I want, what do I see about their behaviors and how they carry themselves, about their actions? I care about their actions, not that they talk about helping others but that they actually do it. They're not in conflict. They're not suing people. They don't fight. A person in recovery doesn't do that. They're helping people. That's what I want. That's how I define recovery."

—SIXTY-FIVE-YEAR-OLD MAN

"Recovery is an act of love."

—SIXTY-YEAR-OLD MAN

"When I first got sober, I got the impression that AA is the same as recovery, but it isn't. Recovery is so much more."

—FIFTY-YEAR-OLD WOMAN

"Today, my children have a mother, my school has a scholar, and my community has an activist. Tonight, I will get my children from daycare, take them home, get them dinner on time, help them finish their homework, and put them to bed. Recovery means I got to wake up this morning and live God's will for me."

—THIRTY-YEAR-OLD WOMAN

"After three years in the recovery community, I don't think of myself as being in recovery anymore. I don't want the label. I'm just me."

—FIFTY-YEAR-OLD MAN

"At first, it was about changing my ways, not lying, not using drugs or alcohol, getting a job. Slowly, over time, it became much bigger than that. It's a whole 360 thing. It's about finding purpose, connection, common ground. Being more understanding and compassionate. It's got a lot to do with empathy. I feel like I'm getting more and more into my recovery the more empathetic I become as a person. It's not necessarily about drugs and alcohol anymore, which is crazy."

—THIRTY-FIVE-YEAR-OLD MAN

"Recovery means creating a better life for myself, my family, and ultimately my community. When I find recovery, everything around me also finds recovery."

—FORTY-YEAR-OLD MAN

"Recovery means everything to me."

—FORTY-FIVE-YEAR-OLD MAN

I have talked with scores of people about their recovery from addiction since I began conducting interviews and focus groups in 2013. I've interviewed family members of people in recovery and attended their support groups to learn about their experiences living with addiction in their families and supporting the people they love seeking recovery. I've interviewed clinicians and leading researchers and read countless academic articles and opinion pieces in my quest to define and thoroughly understand recovery. In all this searching for the answer to "What is recovery?" I concluded that there's simply no single answer. It's impossible to describe the full range of recovery experiences. But there is some common ground.

Narratives from people in all stages of recovery are about incremental changes that add up to people transforming their lives. Some people believe this process starts the moment they stop putting drugs and/or alcohol into their system. Others believe the process begins during active use, when a person starts to think about living differently and may use less, less often, or in a safer way. In any case, people use different strategies along the way to foster change.

Recovery is about more than stopping using substances. It's about repairing the damage done during periods of use, like broken relationships and financial messes, and actively managing emotional and psychological aspects of life that may have been the source of pain and addiction. It's about living a meaningful, healthy life within whatever limitations life plunks down. Recovery isn't linear, and sometimes it can feel like one step forward, two back, and then even more backward. But really, how *could* it be linear? It involves changing and continuing to change *every aspect of life*—mind, body, spirit, family, and community. It's an enormous task, and setbacks are an inevitable part of the process.

In their recovery stories, people describe gaining new perspectives and insights, stepping into new social roles, finding a new community, understanding past trauma, continuing to struggle with mental health, and creating new and deeper relationships. Some of the narratives are uplifting, and others are raw and painful because the new life in recovery is filled with the aftereffects of incarceration, trauma, or psychiatric medications. Some stories have happy endings, and others don't. Taken together, they reveal the individualized nature of recovery. Every person's story is different.

I don't claim to describe the full gamut of these recovery experiences. Among other things, I use the stories people have told me to demonstrate the humility, persistence, courage, and desire to change that we can learn from them. I use them to illustrate the anger and passion that drive their advocacy to make communities better places for people who use drugs and for people in recovery. I hope these stories will convince community members that we can walk alongside people in recovery, grow, and change with them even if they've hurt us, embarrassed us, or let us down in the past. Together, we have the power to create recovery-friendly communities that appreciate everyone's journeys and where the conditions for hope, meaning, healing, and connection can flourish.

When I Say "Recovery," What Comes to Mind?

After introductions and an icebreaker exercise at the beginning of the focus groups I conducted, I asked the question, "When I say 'recovery,' what comes to mind?" The answers supported what researchers are learning about various recovery experiences, ranging from the existential aspect of recovery—just being alive—to feelings of freedom, peace, hope, and gratitude. Other answers were about spending time with family; living life according to core values and morals; experiencing self-awareness and clarity; being part of a community and society; having post-addiction opportunities and possibilities; feeling relief from agony, disgust, and the everyday fight to find drugs and something to eat; and having humility about being given a second or third or fourth chance.

As these responses show, the focus in recovery isn't exclusively abstinence or sobriety. This may come as a surprise to some readers. For most people in recovery, abstinence is an essential first step, but it's not the end goal. It's a means to an end. Abstinence is a way to get to the larger goals of repairing and improving family and social relationships and other areas of life that were dismal and negatively impacted by substance use. Abstinence and recovery usually go hand in hand, but they aren't the same thing. Some people continue to use while they engage in this process of change, and some people stop using substances and never work on changing other aspects of their lives. Ultimately, recovery is best when it focuses on creating the life you want and not just the absence of drugs or alcohol.

Most people I talk with describe recovery as a journey and process, and not a destination. They may not know where they're going, and they're developing the road map along the way, but they're heading toward a new life. Some people refer to "getting well" rather than "being in recovery," acknowledging addiction as a disease and the sickness they felt when substance use dominated their lives. Some say they're "recovered," meaning that their problems with drugs and alcohol are over, and they're living a different life.[1] Others avoid the word "recovery" altogether because it implies going back to a dangerous and dark place that created the conditions of their addiction.

Responses show that recovery isn't just about the individual's journey; family and other relationships are at the heart of this healing process. Addiction can hit a family like a hurricane, and recovering from that takes time and hard work. Some families never make their way out of the rubble. The people in recovery that I spoke with appreciated the relatives and friends who helped them and understood their own responsibilities in improving relationships. "Recovery is when you love someone enough to make changes for them," one person said, a statement that applies equally to the person in recovery, close family members, and other loved ones.

A new sense of self, purpose, and empowerment is a standard part of most stories. Faye told me how empowered she felt when she learned about what she had to offer in the community. "I had a radical spiritual experience. I felt shame at a cellular level and was filled with self-loathing, and I went from that to finding that I could help other women. People outside the recovery community don't understand the importance of giving back. It's really about feeling useful. Gratitude gets you to that place, but what keeps you there is going from feeling useless to understanding that your experience has value and feeling like you are of use."

Recovery Identity

One typical recovery trajectory is to stop using substances, create a new identity and new social networks in the recovery community, and then integrate into the broader community. Alcoholics Anonymous (AA) is often the starting point because it's widely available, free, and forms the core of many treatment programs. The 12-step program is a road map that helps many people get started, and being a part of it is instrumental for many in creating their new recovery identity and social networks. The founders of AA developed a narrative style about addiction and recovery that helps people find that new identity by hearing stories they can relate to. People "in the rooms" share "the way things were while I was drinking, what happened when I stopped, and the way things are now." They also share their "experience, strength, and hopes" to demonstrate that recovery is possible for the newcomer. Some people start in AA and stay "in the program" the rest of their lives. They peg a core part of their identity on being a member of AA, being in recovery, and telling their story over and over. Others begin their journey in AA and then move on, accepting their AA identity as part of their past. Still others who start with AA find that the narrative doesn't reflect their own experience, and they reject it as useless or harmful to their process of change.

Not everyone who has resolved a drug or alcohol problem considers themselves in recovery. This is especially true in some ethnic communities. As one middle-aged Latina told me, "My recovery community is a very small part of my life ... being in recovery isn't the important part of my identity." She had a supportive family and network of friends. "So many people like me didn't lose their jobs, didn't lose their families. Things got very bad internally, but they had a lot of recovery capital. Recovery doesn't become their main identity, and they don't need to speak up about it. People who are willing to tell their stories publicly did have that rock bottom experience. But family support, money for treatment, education opportunities—that part of the story is rarely heard."

Asking, "What is recovery?" is like asking, "What is wellness?" People answer the question based on their own experiences, cultural identity, family life, community, spiritual beliefs, aspirations, and more. In the end, recovery is about creating the life you want. To the extent that any of us can determine where our life is going, that is recovery. As the Latina in long-term recovery said, "It is the human experience, rooted in my cultural heritage."

"CLEAN" OR "SOBER" OR "IN RECOVERY"?

Terminology around recovery can be confusing. People in recovery circles talk about being "clean," which means not having any mind-altering substances in the body. In treatment settings, "clean" means not having drugs show up in a urine test. This term has fallen out of favor for many because the opposite is "dirty," which implies that people using drugs are dirty. (But it's not uncommon to hear clinicians refer to people having "dirty" urine when substances show up in a urinalysis.) In 12-step circles, "being clean and sober" means being abstinent and having a healthy spiritual, emotional, and social life. These days, though, instead of talking about being "clean and sober," many people talk about being in recovery. To confuse matters further, some people use "sober" or "living in sobriety" to mean just abstaining from drugs or alcohol but not also engaging in the transformative and healing process of recovery.

Who Is in Recovery?

Andrew moved to Portland, Maine, to live in a recovery residence and for several years after that, he made his life there. In recovery circles, Portland has a reputation for being a "recovery town" because of its many recovery support services. Treatment agencies from around the country recommend living in a Portland recovery residence as part of recovery plans. The city is a destination for people of all ages in early recovery, but especially young people. One woman in early recovery summed it up this way: "Portland is a 'young people' recovery town. People talk about their recovery instead of what happened before that. People talk about how they got over major things while still staying sober, and that gives us hope that we can do it, too."

Like many of the people in recovery in Portland, Andrew is in his thirties, white, and from a family with the financial means to support residential treatment and living in a recovery residence afterward. This image of people in recovery—young, privileged, white—captured the media's attention in the early 2010s, when opioid overdose deaths started to rise sharply among white people, and an acceptable addiction and recovery story was born. The press latched onto stories about young white people, usually from the suburbs or rural areas, who became innocently addicted to pre- scribed painkillers (opioids) after taking them for legitimate pain, and their stories underscored the notion that "addiction can happen to anyone."[2,3] Indeed, "anyone can become addicted" is a tagline for some treatment agen- cies and for the National Institute on Drug Abuse, and it's the rallying cry for the New Recovery Advocacy Movement.

The truth is that the most widely used and deadliest drug (excluding nic- otine) remains alcohol, not opioids, and addiction isn't an equal opportunity disease. It strikes people of color and populations with low incomes at much higher rates than white communities.[4,5] Recovery, like addiction, also doesn't happen on an even playing field. Some people have a smoother time of it than others. Parents with means can pay for treatment, support services, and edu- cation after treatment. They're often well connected to possible employment opportunities, too. Because alcohol is a legal drug, people in recovery from alcohol use disorder don't have to face the consequences of having committed crimes by using it. The same is true for people in states where cannabis is legal. When illegal substances are involved, people with financial means can afford attorneys who help them avoid the criminal justice system if they have commit- ted criminal offenses. People with felony convictions live with their records their entire lives, creating enormous challenges for finding safe housing, meaningful employment, and education. People of color are incarcerated for drug-related offenses at higher rates than white people, which has had a tremendous impact on their futures and communities.[6] Women have different recovery experiences than men, often because they have added responsibilities of taking care of chil- dren or may have lost custody of their children during active use.

Sometimes people don't say they're in recovery because it's not safe. For example, "coming out" as a person in recovery who also identifies as LGBTQIA+ (lesbian, gay, bisexual, trans, queer, intersex, asexual, and others) can layer stigma on top of stigma and create additional risk for exclusion or violence.

The media has adopted one recovery story based on the AA narrative: People move from living "the life" of using drugs to a conventional lifestyle that includes work, family, and good health. It's impossible to overstate the importance of people standing up in public and telling their stories. They change lives. But it's critical to recognize that not all recovery stories follow this storyline. If you dig deeper, you might find that some people chose a life of using drugs as an act of disobedience and rebellion in a world that didn't accept who they were. In recovery, they're still not interested in conforming to a conventional lifestyle. You might also find that life after addiction isn't always all good. Past trauma and grappling with mental illness and the after-effects of psychiatric medications all have an enormous impact in some people's lives in recovery and don't disappear once they stop using drugs.

What Can Allies Do?

The bottom line is that recovery isn't the same for everyone. If you want to know what recovery is like, you have to ask. And then you have to listen.

For Everyone

- Explore your attitudes toward recovery. What is your definition? Is it consistent with what people in recovery say? Do you think abstinence is the same as recovery?

- What experiences have you had with people in recovery? Does knowing they are in recovery change the way you think about them? What have you learned from them about recovery? Where could you learn more about recovery in your community?

- Consider starting a conversation about recovery with your colleagues, neighbors, or family members. Create a safe space for people to ask questions and learn about recovery.

For Friends and Family Members

- Ask your loved ones what recovery means to them and spend some time learning from them. They may not want to use the word "recovery," but maybe they'll talk about what they want from life now that they have decided to cut back on or not use drugs or alcohol. If they're open to a conversation, ask them how you can support them.

- If their recovery story isn't perfect, if it is full of pain and challenge, don't brush that under the rug by saying something like "Well, at least you aren't using drugs anymore." Recovery is about living a full life, not just about abstinence. If you accept that they are having a hard time finding that full life, they might be able to tell you something specific you can do to make their journey easier.

- Individual resilience can help prevent a minor setback from turning into a full-blown return to substance use. Families can be resilient, too, by adapting and figuring out together how to thrive when so much change, including setbacks, is happening. Talk about stressful events in your lives and brainstorm about how to improve the ways you deal with them.

- If your loved one isn't open to conversation, find ways to spend time with them that don't involve talking about "it" (their recovery)— just try to create positive connections if they're open to them.

For Health Care Providers, Social Workers, and Clergy

- Service providers and clergy are in important positions to be strong allies. If you have patients, clients, or congregation members who are in recovery, ask them what their recovery means to them and if it's OK to help them look for resources to support them. Be willing to accept their path, even if it's not the one you think is best for them. Linking them with peers is especially important. Ask if their families need anything, and find resources for them, too.

RECOVERY RESEARCH

PEOPLE IN RECOVERY see their recovery from the inside, close up, and understand what works for them. They're the experts in their own recovery. But there's a difference between the personal experience of one individual and a broader understanding of recovery based on science and research. Recovery as a process of improving health and wellness, growing, learning, and reaching one's full potential varies considerably from one person to the next, at different points in time, and in diverse social contexts. Understanding this from a scientific perspective is challenging. One researcher aptly referred to recovery as "an overloaded container concept," with its many dimensions yet to be understood from a research perspective.[1]

Researchers know that what works for one person doesn't necessarily work for all, but they have shown some commonalities:

- Recovery support services, education, employment, and housing are critical factors in early recovery, and social support—including family and community support—aids recovery at all stages.

- The amount of recovery capital people have—all of the assets they bring to their recovery—is a good predictor of sustained recovery.

- Another good predictor of recovery is a successful shift to a network of people who don't use drugs or alcohol and a change in identity to a person who doesn't use.

- Sustained recovery is the norm, although pathways and time to initiate recovery vary from one person to the next.

- Barriers to recovery include mental health issues, access to treatment and other services, self-esteem, stigma, and social isolation.

- When it comes to treatment and recovery, continuity of care and linking to recovery support services as soon as possible lead to better results.

Turning to research doesn't mean ignoring or discounting individual healing experiences and their power as examples for others seeking recovery. It also doesn't mean promoting evidence-based practices at the expense of successes that haven't yet been studied. It's just to say that if we are to gain broader support for recovery-friendly communities and expand connections with people in recovery, there are questions that research can help answer.

A Uniform Definition of Recovery

In the past twenty years, organizations and researchers have developed definitions of recovery, usually based on a panel comprising people in recovery, researchers, and policy experts who reach a consensus definition. Several such consensus definitions exist.[2] The Substance Abuse and Mental Health Services Administration (SAMHSA), the nation's largest public funder of substance use and mental health projects, created a "working definition" that is most often used. Its definition of recovery, which guides federal policy, is "a process of change through which individuals improve their health and wellness, live a self-directed life, and strive to reach their full potential."[3]

This definition doesn't include what has traditionally been a requirement of recovery: abstinence from all mind-altering drugs and alcohol. Instead, it allows for a broader view that focuses on self-defined criteria that may or may not include abstinence. In recent years, harm reductionists have taken this to heart and started conversations about harm reduction as a part of the recovery journey, thereby blurring the lines between harm reduction and recovery. The result is a new challenge to advocacy efforts to explain how these two conditions—using drugs and being in recovery—can co-exist.

Recovery researchers needed a definition to move their research forward, but it wasn't just for them. Defining recovery can have tremendous real-life consequences. For example, it may determine who retains custody of their children. One woman I know, who has been in recovery for more than five years and regained custody of her children four years ago, recently received a call from the state's child protective services agency to require her to take a urine test. The agency requires abstinence from all substances for her to retain custody, and a neighbor had spotted her "looking like she was high." The urine test was negative for all psychoactive substances.

Measuring Recovery

Researchers have no consistent way to measure recovery.[4] Until recently, recovery research focused on individual outcomes of people in residential treatment or counseling settings where abstinence is the primary outcome. Family engagement, employment, and other measures of healing and wellness, as well as quality of life, were secondary outcomes. This approach ensured that researchers learned about people with severe problems and probably mental health issues, but not much about other people. That left out the vast number of people who recover without treatment, either by choice or because they lack access to it. Researchers rarely focused on outcomes beyond six months or a year, so they learned little about long-term recovery. Current research focuses on measuring of recovery capital to document the process of change in recovery rather than treatment outcomes. (See chapter 5: Recovery Capital: All That People Bring to Their Recovery.)

Recovery by the Numbers

People in recovery are living in plain sight, and yet we don't see them. Some people are vocal about their recovery and are active in advocacy work. However, these people are the tip of the recovery iceberg. Everyone else is virtually invisible.

Estimates of the number of Americans in recovery vary because, as we've seen, there's no agreed-on definition. Also, we have no record-keeping system for diagnoses of addiction or recovery from drugs or alcohol. The estimates we have are based on self-reported survey responses about remission from symptoms of a substance use disorder (remission is when a person hasn't met diagnosable criteria for the past year) and scientific studies of specific groups who have received treatment. Marginalized groups, including people of color, people without housing, and people living in jails and prisons, are typically underrepresented in these surveys and studies. So, we know very little about them. Estimates are that 5.3–15.3 percent of the US adult population is in recovery from a mild, moderate, or severe substance use disorder.[5] Leading recovery advocacy organizations like Faces and Voices of Recovery rely on estimates to claim that about 23 million people are in recovery from substance use disorder (mild, moderate, or severe) in the United States today.[6]

To make matters even more complicated, not everyone who fits the definition of being in recovery thinks of themselves that way. People with mild substance use disorders that resolved generally don't consider themselves in recovery. In the National Recovery Survey, the first national probability-based sample of US adults who self-identify as having resolved a significant alcohol or drug problem, slightly fewer than half (46 percent), or 10.7 million, identified themselves as being in recovery.[7]

The Stages of Change and Stages of Recovery

Researchers have developed models to understand how people move from using drugs or alcohol to early recovery to sustained recovery. The **Transtheoretical Stages of Change Model** is a well-established theory of behavior change that addiction professionals apply in treatment settings and peers use when they provide recovery support services.[8] People who have engaged in counseling for behavior change, weight loss, or smoking cessation will be familiar with this widely used model. In a nutshell, the theory posits that there are five stages of change that people go through when they are considering a behavior change, including entering and sustaining recovery. Effectively supporting a person's change means understanding their "stage of change" to give them the support that best aligns with that stage.

In the context of substance use, in the *precontemplative stage,* a person isn't aware of the problems associated with their substance use, and they're resistant to any type of intervention or help. Harm reduction services are vital in this stage. In the *contemplative stage,* a person is aware of the problem but doesn't know what to do. They're open to learning more, and it may be helpful to provide them with information about treatment options and recovery services. In the *preparation stage,* the person accepts responsibility for their behavior and takes steps to make changes. Here, it may be helpful to talk about the pros and cons of their current behavior to help tip the balance toward change. In the *action stage,* the person consciously and enthusiastically chooses new behaviors and gains new insights and skills. People in this stage are often open to discussions about strategies and activities to change their behavior. Finally, in the *maintenance stage,* a person has mastered the ability to maintain recovery, has less frequent urges to use, and focuses on avoiding relapses.

Figure 4.1 describes each stage of change and related treatment and recovery support services.[9]

Beyond the maintenance stage of change, sustained recovery begins. There are several models for **stages of recovery** that use different time frames for each stage.[10] Generally, the stages start with stabilization in *early recovery,* when the body and the brain are cleared of substances, and life circumstances like housing and relationships begin to improve. In *middle recovery,* people repair relationships with families and friends and make lifestyle choices that allow them to pursue life goals, like getting an education, advancing a career, or pursuing spiritual goals. They begin to see an integration of their personal values and outward actions. In *late recovery,* people resolve long-standing emotional difficulties from childhood and other life experiences, allowing them to deepen their relationships. Finally, in *long-term recovery,* usually after five years of sustained recovery, people may experience life fulfillment.

Figure 4.1. Stages of Change and Related Treatment and Recovery Support Services

PRECONTEMPLATIVE	CONTEMPLATIVE	PREPARATION	ACTION	MAINTENANCE
In this stage, individuals are not even thinking about changing their behavior. They do not see their addiction as a problem: they often think others who point out the problem are exaggerating.	In this stage, people are more aware of the personal consequences of their addiction and spend time thinking about their problem. Although they are able to consider the possibility of changing, they tend to be ambivalent about it.	In this stage, people have made a commitment to make a change. This stage involves information gathering about what they will need to change their behavior.	In this stage, individuals believe they have the ability to change their behavior and actively take steps to change their behavior.	In this stage, individuals maintain their sobriety, successfully avoiding temptations and relapse.

HARM REDUCTION
- Emergency Services (i.e., Narcan)
- Needle Exchanges
- Supervised Injection Sites

SCREENING AND FEEDBACK
- Brief Advice
- Motivational Interventions

SCREENING, BRIEF INTERVENTION, AND REFERRAL TO TREATMENT (SBIRT)

CLINICAL INTERVENTION
- Phases/Levels (e.g., inpatient, residential, outpatient)
- Intervention Types
  - Psychosocial (e.g., Cognitive Behavioral Therapy)
  - Medications: Agonists (e.g., Buprenorphine, Methadone) and Antagonists (Naltrexone)

NONCLINICAL INTERVENTION
- Self-Management/Natural Recovery (e.g., self-help books, online resources)
- Mutual Help Organizations (e.g., Alcoholics Anonymous, SMART Recovery, LifeRing Secular Recovery)
- Community Support Services (e.g., Recovery Community Centers, Recovery Ministries, Recovery Employment Assistance)

CONTINUING CARE (3 months–1 year)
Recovery Management Checkups, Telephone Counseling, Mobile Applications, Text Message Interventions

RECOVERY MONITORING (1–5+ years)
Continued Recovery Management Checkups, Therapy Visits, Primary Care Provider Visits

Source: Adapted with permission by Recovery Research Institute, Massachusetts General Hospital, RecoveryAnswers.org.

Emerging Trends in Recovery Research

Researchers are just beginning to explore not only treatment and what supports early and sustained recovery, but *how* those supports work. Research topics include:

- If recovery is about connecting and reconnecting with one's broader community in a meaningful way, how does this happen?

- Are different types of connections significant at different stages of recovery?

- If hope and gratitude are critical, as so many people in recovery tell us, how do they work, and how can we promote them?

- If recovery support services help sustain recovery, what's the best way to put them in place in the community?

- How do we measure a person's recovery from one substance if they are still using another?

Trailblazing researchers like Dr. John Kelly at Harvard University, Dr. Keith Humphreys at Stanford University, Dr. David Best at the University of Derby, and their research teams are expanding our knowledge about recovery by leaps and bounds. William L. White, now retired, has contributed hundreds of research articles, blogs, and books about recovery and remains active in recovery research. These and other researchers are taking our understandings to the next level and are working on some of the following topics.

Defining Success

If recovery is a process of change, how do we define success? Most research to date has used the length of time in abstinence as a critical indicator of success, which doesn't align with a definition of recovery as a process of change. "How many [sober] days do you have?" is a common question in the recovery community. Yet, this focus on abstinence obscures the fact that a return to use is often a critical learning experience instead of a failure that sets the recovery clock back to zero. "Progress, not perfection" is an often-heard comment when someone has a slip. Focusing on abstinence also obscures the reality that many people in recovery use substances recreationally. Some researchers have moved away from abstinence as the sole measure of success and are looking at quality-of-life measures.[11]

Unit of Measure

Research has focused predominantly on individuals in recovery and family therapy to help families heal. Still, we know that addiction is detrimental to the community as well. Some research has shown that increasing the number of people in recovery is good for the community where they live by reducing crime and increasing community engagement through employment, education, and volunteerism.[12] We need to know more about the ripple effects that individual and family recovery have on the community.

Specific Groups

We've seen that not all people recover the same way, so research should reflect this.[13] Research should be directed to understanding the different recovery pathways and needs for recovery support services for women, men, veterans, immigrant groups, people in the LGBTQIA+ community, people of color, and others. More participatory research—a method that brings researchers and the "target community" together to develop the research topics and project design—could be effective here. Community members often combine participatory research with community outreach, education, and political action. For example, bringing trans people in recovery and recovery residence managers for a participatory research project could lead the way to create best practices for recovery housing for trans people.

The Recovery Timeline

Even though researchers think of substance use disorder as chronic, they typically research only the early stages of recovery. Recovery capital and supports vary at different stages of recovery. We need to understand what resources need to be in place so that people in recovery have the help they need for sustained recovery for up to five years. (At five years, the chance of returning to use is considered 15 percent, the remission marker for other diseases.[14])

Recovery Support Services

Researchers have long understood the importance of support services, such as peer support, especially in early recovery. Now they're exploring in more detail, for example, what "essential ingredients" a recovery community center needs to be effective.[15] Similarly, research on recovery residences is positive, but we need to know more about those essential ingredients for recovery housing. Also, we need research to better understand how health care systems can integrate peer support services into their broader care system for people in recovery.[16]

Impact of Public Policies on the Recovery Community

Public policies directed toward other aspects of substance use, like prevention and treatment, can have tremendous implications for the recovery community. For example,

- We know that the younger a person starts using substances, the greater the likelihood of developing a severe substance use problem, and the age of first use has been worrisomely declining for many years. Ineffective policies directed toward preventing youth substance use may result in younger people entering recovery. Treatment programs and recovery support services developed for adults may not meet their needs.

- The impact of policies to increase access to medications for opioid addiction—by, for example, increasing Medicaid reimbursement rates—may result in more people receiving treatment, thereby increasing the need for recovery support services.

- Investigating policy changes during the COVID-19 pandemic, which made virtual counseling for substance use and peer recovery support possible, may show that this method is effective in helping people sustain their recovery. Research can show us who benefits from virtual support and who prefers in-person support.

What Can Allies Do?

Recovery research is in its infancy, so there's a lot we don't know. Don't believe everything you read! There's a lot of money to be made in addiction treatment and recovery, and for-profit providers and others have a financial interest in making you believe that what they do "works." Before you jump in with both feet, spend some time learning what the experts have to say.

The Recovery Research Institute of Massachusetts General Hospital (an affiliate of Harvard Medical School) is a tremendous resource, free of charge, to anyone with an internet connection. The institute is made up of prominent recovery researchers and practitioners dedicated to advancing addiction treatment and recovery. Professionals at the institute review research and explain it in simple terms as well as in technical language. Each review includes the "Bottom Line" for individuals and families seeking recovery, scientists, policy makers, treatment professionals, and treatment systems. The Recovery Research Institute is online at www.recoveryanswers.org.

SECTION 2
Recovery-Friendly Communities

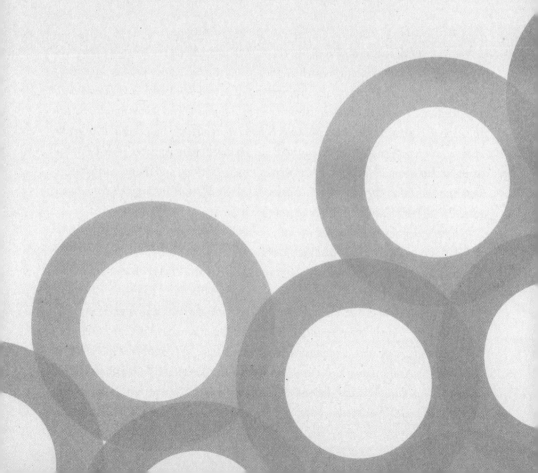

5

RECOVERY CAPITAL:
ALL THAT PEOPLE BRING
TO THEIR RECOVERY

FAYE IS FROM Seattle and now lives in a small town along the coast of Maine. As a child, she lived in a chaotic household that included drugs, and she was repeatedly sexually abused. At fourteen, she dropped out of school, left home, and moved onto the streets, where she felt safer and more accepted than she had in her family. By the time she was sixteen, her drug use was beyond her control. "I was unable to make choices for myself, and it was so painful. I got a moment of relief when I used, but the torment that went with it was far greater." The self-loathing and shame she felt were so tremendous that she used drugs to destroy herself. She had no support around her to deal with her childhood trauma in another way.

In her twenties, Faye moved in with her aunt, a university professor who provided a safe place to live, helped her develop her reading skills, asked her to share household responsibilities, and took her to cultural events. "It was an amazing experience to go from being in the gutter to being embraced like that," Faye said. "My aunt looked past the ugliness of addiction to see the truth of me as a person. It was like my aunt said, 'I know your beauty, and you're not going to convince me otherwise.' What she did for me was way more helpful than anything I got in treatment."

Over the years, Faye had been on medications for ADHD (attention-deficit/hyperactivity disorder) and depression, but they never had the results they were supposed to have. "I wanted so badly to be a functional member of society," she said.

"I wanted to be normal with all my heart, but it didn't happen." When she learned about complex trauma and its effects on brain development—it's a brain injury that impacts every aspect of her life—she started to understand her life in a different light.

In her thirties now, Faye feels there's only one way that a person is considered a functional contributor in our society, and that's to get an education and have a job. That's a problem. "I finally understand that I have value. All that I have survived has innate, tremendous value, and yet I'll probably never be able to get a college degree. I can't retain information the way our society wants us to, but you put me in front of a girl that has trauma the way I did, and I know that I can be at least as helpful for her as someone with a master's degree. I know that. And yet there's no room for that in the workforce."

Faye has moved out of the AA community, where she found powerful experiences helping other women but little support for dealing with trauma. Now she doesn't know how to be helpful. "It's my heart's desire, and I want more than anything to be able to do that. I don't know where to do it." What can community members do to support a recovery path like hers? "Create space for life experience to be of value to the community—bring in people with diverse experiences and find a place for us. We want to be useful. It may be more expensive and take more time than a quick fix, but then you have the reward of this rich soul that has been returned to wholeness and is a contributing member of society. The thought that I could be useful to someone was just radical! I would do anything to be useful."

Ron grew up in a suburb of Philadelphia and went to medical school right after college. When his family first found out about his drug use, which had gotten out of control during residency training, they were shocked. "They didn't see it coming," Ron says. His parents, especially his mother, were very supportive. They were non-judgmental and sent a clear message to him: "We love our son, no matter what." They educated themselves about opioid addiction. While Ron went to Alcoholics Anonymous and Narcotics Anonymous meetings, his mother started a Narcotics Anonymous group in her town in Florida. "They helped themselves with their own issues honestly, and that helped me to be honest with them, so I could tell them when I was safe and when they needed to worry."

Ron got his medical license and practiced medicine. He had long periods of sobriety interspersed with short periods of using. Eventually, he lost his license because of his use and participated in the Washington Physicians Health Program (WPHP) for

sixteen years. Most of the people in the program were like him, Ron explains. "They had
a fair amount of recovery capital already, like a safe home, a supportive family, money,
and transportation, to name a few." To participate in the program, WPHP participants
have to agree to urine screens and go to AA meetings and counseling in an environment
of peer support. In return, the program provides case managers. In Ron's case, the pro-
gram advocated for him before the medical board, which reinstated his license.

Ron always had support from many of his friends, and most kept in contact no
matter what. He made sure he kept them in the loop about how he was doing, and
they took his phone calls and sent letters when he was in treatment or prison, or
wherever. "My friends sent the message 'We're not betraying you. We're not rejecting
you. We care about you and want you to be part of our lives.' There wasn't a cold
wind when I reached out to them. You find out who your friends are, and it's not
always who you expect." One of his best friends, though, didn't understand addiction
and rejected him. The relationship was damaged and never recovered. For Ron, it
remains a painful memory.

After a career that included directing a methadone clinic, running a company
that provided drug-free workplace program services to industry, and working for
a company that created and sold electronic medical records software, and after a
relapse that resulted in additional treatment and living in a recovery residence,
Ron retired and is now actively engaged in Portland, Maine's recovery community.
He directs the Maine Association of Recovery Residences, which certifies quality
recovery residences, and supports legislative initiatives that create harm reduction
programs and recovery support services in the state.

The differences in these two recovery stories are stark. Ron came from a
financially secure and emotionally supportive family and was an educated
physician when he started his recovery journey. Faye's upbringing was chaotic
and filled with trauma, then homelessness. Both are in long-term recovery
now, but Faye had far fewer resources to support her recovery than Ron. With
less recovery capital to work with—generally speaking, all the assets she was
able to bring to her recovery—her path has been much bumpier.

Cultivating This Capital

As community members, we play a tremendous role in creating a place where
the recovery path is smoother, and recovery can flourish. This is what I've

been referring to as a "recovery-friendly community."[1] As individuals, we can be supportive of and compassionate to people in recovery, but there's more we can do collectively. As a community, we can create physical, cultural, and social environments that are conducive to sustained recovery. We can create the community "scaffolding" for individuals to heal and grow.[2] A public health approach to recovery relies heavily on the concept of recovery capital and creating recovery capital, which is the most important activity that we can do to help people in recovery and their families heal and move ahead in their lives. When communities take this on, working seriously to become recovery friendly, they benefit from a larger and healthier workforce, healthy parents, engaged students, reduced crime, and more.

Research

What do we need for a healthy life? Safe housing, food, and clothing. Physical and emotional safety, health and wellness, and financial security. Friendships, intimacy, a sense of belonging. Self-esteem. A sense of purpose, hope, goals in life. Spiritual contentment. These are the building blocks of a meaningful life. How do people in recovery attain these? That's where recovery capital comes in. Researchers have conducted studies to understand what resources people need to initiate and maintain wellness, and they developed the concept of recovery capital. They have found that generally speaking, the more recovery capital a person has, the better their chances of sustained recovery.[3]

Researchers, counselors, and people in recovery have learned quite a bit about recovery capital since the term first came into use.[4,5] Researchers looked at different ways to define recovery capital and ways to measure it. Boiled down to the essentials, here are its various components:

- *Personal recovery capital* means the characteristics and capabilities of the person seeking and in recovery, like knowledge, communication, interpersonal skills, coping skills, mental health, problem-solving skills, self-esteem, resilience, and hope. Personal recovery capital also includes tangible resources like safe housing; food; transportation; money and financial stability; insurance; and personal beliefs, values, preferences, and behavior that come with belonging to a particular cultural group.

- *Social recovery capital* refers to supportive social relationships and networks in the recovery community and the broader community, supportive family relationships, and connections with social institutions like a faith community.

- *Community capital* is the resources available in the broader community that support recovery, including evidence-based treatment, support services like recovery community centers, and housing policies that don't discriminate against recovery residences. Community capital also has to do with the attitudes of community members and their openness to fully welcome people in recovery.

This last point is crucial: stable and sustained community participation can't be the individual's responsibility alone. It requires family and community involvement in interpersonal relationships, and it requires people like business owners, librarians, university deans and professors, landlords, bankers, law enforcement officers, construction contractors, childcare providers, teachers and school administrators, doctors, dentists, fitness instructors, and so many more to maintain opportunities for people to participate in community life again. It requires policies and cultural norms that create and support these opportunities for people to get their lives back on track.

Measuring Recovery Capital

Researchers and practitioners have developed different tools to assess a person's recovery capital. People in recovery use the results of their assessment to establish their individual recovery plans. The assessment can be administered periodically, every three months, for example, at recovery residences, in recovery community centers, or during long-term treatment to track changes in recovery capital.

One commonly used assessment is the Recovery Capital Scale developed by William White and published in 2009.[6] Treatment providers often use the assessment to determine areas of need at discharge. Individuals in recovery use it to track their progress.

Recovery Capital Scale

Place a number by each statement that best summarizes your situation.

5. Strongly Agree

4. Agree

3. Sometimes

2. Disagree

1. Strongly Disagree

___ I have the financial resources to provide for myself and my family.

___ I have personal transportation or access to public transportation.

___ I live in a home and neighborhood that is safe and secure.

___ I live in an environment free from alcohol and other drugs.

___ I have an intimate partner supportive of my recovery process.

___ I have family members who are supportive of my recovery process.

___ I have friends who are supportive of my recovery process.

___ I have people close to me (intimate partner, family members, or friends) who are also in recovery.

___ I have a stable job that I enjoy and that provides for my basic necessities.

___ I have an education or work environment that is conducive to my long-term recovery.

___ I continue to participate in a continuing care program of an addiction treatment program (e.g., groups, alumni association meetings, etc.).

___ I have a professional assistance program that is monitoring and supporting my recovery process.

___ I have a primary care physician who attends to my health problems.

___ I am now in reasonably good health.

___ I have an active plan to manage any lingering or potential health problems.

___ I am on prescribed medication that minimizes my cravings for alcohol and other drugs.

___ I have insurance that will allow me to receive help for major health problems.

___ I have access to regular, nutritious meals.

___ I have clothes that are comfortable, clean, and conducive to my recovery activities.

___ I have access to recovery support groups in my local community.

___ I have established close affiliation with a local recovery support group.

___ I have a sponsor (or equivalent) who serves as a special mentor related to my recovery.

___ I have access to online recovery support groups.

___ I have completed or am complying with all legal requirements related to my past.

___ There are other people who rely on me to support their own recoveries.

___ My immediate physical environment contains literature, tokens, posters, or other symbols of my commitment to recovery.

___ I have recovery rituals that are now part of my daily life.

___ I had a profound experience that marked the beginning or deepening of my commitment to recovery.

___ I now have goals and great hopes for my future.

___ I have problem-solving skills and resources that I lacked during my years of active addiction.

___ I feel like I have meaningful, positive participation in my family and community.

___ Today I have a clear sense of who I am.

___ I know that my life has a purpose.

___ Service to others is now an important part of my life.

___ My personal values and sense of right and wrong have become clearer and stronger in recent years.

Possible Score: 175

My Score: _____

The areas in which I scored lowest were the following:

1. _____

2. _____

3. _____

4. _____

5. _____

Recovery Capital Plan

After completing and reviewing the Recovery Capital Scale, complete the following.

In the next year, I will increase my recovery capital by doing the following:

Goal #1: _____

Goal #2: _____

Goal #3: _____

Goal #4: _____

My Recovery Capital "To Do" List

In the next week, I will do the following activities to move closer to achieving the above goals:

1. _____

2. _____

3. _____

4. _____

5. _____

Recovery Capital and Social Justice

Not every community has the same resources to support recovery, and people in "recovery deserts," where few supports exist, may find it difficult to enter and maintain recovery. Addiction and isolation happen everywhere—in urban areas and rural areas—but low-income communities are especially hard hit and challenged in being recovery friendly. Financial resources are an important aspect of creating recovery capital, but if we keep in mind that recovery equals connection, we can figure out ways to develop a supportive community anywhere.

Original recovery capital research conducted by Robert Granfield and William Cloud in 1999 focused predominantly on white male adults in early, natural recovery (without treatment or other external support), whose goals were to lead a conventional lifestyle. Education, employment, and stable relationships were a critical part of their recovery, and poverty and incarceration were not part of their stories.[7] But we know that recovery capital isn't distributed equally: Some communities have more wealth, social cohesion, programs, and services than others and will have an easier road to becoming recovery friendly. Our history of racial segregation and mass incarceration and the ripple effects in communities of color are key reasons for reduced recovery capital in those communities.[8] Economic shifts, with our manufacturing jobs exported overseas, have left other communities impoverished and with frail local economies unable to support their citizens. Researchers are just beginning to look at recovery capital in minority groups, among people who don't want a conventional lifestyle in recovery, and in marginalized groups, such as people who are experiencing homelessness. For now, we have little scientific knowledge about building recovery capital in these communities.[9]

A New Conversation

I believe it's time to shift our conversation about addiction and recovery from what's wrong (deficits) to what's working (recovery capital). An important part of recovery is good citizenship. As people's recovery capital increases, they're better able to build new networks and find new meaning in life. That's far easier in an environment rich in community capital. They can engage in a civic life of shared values and commitments, networks, and relationships—these are the things that expand a community's recovery capital. People in recovery can become positive forces and contributors to the broader community. They can shift from drawing on community resources to making active contributions to the community, which in turn creates a healthier community for the next person in recovery.[10, 11] As William White says, "Recovery is contagious and passes from one visible carrier to another."[12]

What Can Allies Do?

Our strongest suit as community members is to provide individual support and compassion and then work on building recovery capital in the community by changing community and institutional resources, social norms, and policies.[13] Some of our support is one-on-one, and some of it is collective and supports many people. This doesn't require a lot of money. As recovery researcher David Best said, "Look at community resources, not reimbursable services. Start with people power and whatever assets are available. You can start with a knitting club and grow from there."[14]

The journey to sustained recovery (at least one year) can take people eight or nine years after they first seek formal help,[15] and they need different types of community support throughout that time. A typical trajectory is to quit using substances, create a new identity and new social networks, and then integrate into a broader community. In the first year or so after quitting, people need to have strong peer support and life essentials such as food, clothing, and safe housing. Once they meet their basic needs, they can work to get their finances in order, get back custody of their children, and repair broken relationships. Volunteering and working in the community represent a first step in creating a new identity and new social networks. People at that point are acquiring new skills, looking for work, or going back to school.

For Family Members

- Find ways to support your loved one as a resource in their own recovery by asking them what you can offer or what they need. Support any positive changes they are making toward wellness.

- Create opportunities to share life skills with your family member if they're open to it. For example, try preparing a meal together or sharing childcare responsibilities.

- Make a point of inviting your son or daughter, husband or wife, sister or brother to family gatherings if it's safe to do so. It might be awkward for everyone the first few times, but it's an important step in the family's recovery journey.

- Ask if you can help with transportation, like giving them a ride to work or appointments if they don't have a car or have lost their license. If you live in an area with public transportation, ask if they'd like you to take the bus or subway with them until they feel comfortable doing it independently.

- Support efforts to go back to school, get a job, or volunteer by offering to get more information.

- Take care of yourself so that you have the energy and heart to be nonjudgmental and supportive.

For Everyone

- Examine your attitudes toward recovery. Do you believe a person can be a resource in their own recovery, or do you believe you need to identify their needs for them?

- Make sure you're not using stigmatizing language. Open up a conversation with your friends and family about the best way to talk about recovery so that they're aware, too.

- Be a connector to the recovery community by serving on the board of an agency that serves people in recovery, volunteering at a recovery community center, or helping get one started. Show up at local recovery events like rallies and walks.

For Community Organizations

- Invite people in recovery to serve on your boards, committees, advisory groups, and coalitions. Make sure they're invited as active participants, not token representatives of the recovery community.

- Make sure people in active addiction know that recovery is possible. Examine your organization's communications to be sure this message is included.

- Create volunteer opportunities of all types, and reach out to recovery community centers and recovery residences to connect with volunteers in recovery.

- Create opportunities for community members to learn about recovery through town halls, community meetings, and social media posts. Make sure teachers, coaches, employers, and others know about recovery and how to support people in recovery.

- Make sure support services like recovery community centers, reentry services, and harm reduction services are accessible and integrated into health care services for at least five years beyond the first steps in recovery.

- Make sure recovery support is part of community health coalitions, and engage community leaders to make sure physical, cultural, and social environments are welcoming to people in recovery.

For Health Care Providers

- Ask your patients in recovery what would support their recovery and if they would like you to help them find that support.

- Link with your local recovery community through support groups or recovery community centers, so you know about resources to share with your patients in recovery.

- Learn what services your local health system has to offer for people in recovery, and ask your patients and family members if they would like to be connected with them.[16]

For Policy Makers

- Invite people in recovery to serve on local and state committees and advisory groups that address substance use issues.

- Look at the financing of treatment and recovery support services. Instead of placing most support on the front end of the equation (getting people into treatment), make sure sufficient resources go to where most people are (maintaining recovery).

- Place recovery capital at the center of community values. Make sure funding streams, policies, laws, and systems, such as educational and health care systems, support people at all stages of recovery.

6

BUILDING
RECOVERY-FRIENDLY
COMMUNITIES

"SUPPOSE YOU HAVE a hundred-acre forest, and in that forest, there is a disease or sickness. All the trees are sick. It is a sick forest. Suppose, then, you go to that forest one day, and you take one of those sick trees and temporarily uproot it and put it under your arm. You walk down a road, and you put it in a nursery where there is good soil. Or you take a young person. You take them out of the community and put them in treatment. So now you have this tree in good soil, and it becomes healthy because it is getting sun and rain. It is getting well. It is turning green. You get this tree to be well, and then you take this well tree back to the sick forest. What happens if you take a well tree back to a sick forest? It gets sick again.

"This means that we must actively heal the community and its institutions while individuals work on their healing from alcohol and drugs or other unwell behaviors. The individual affects the community, and the community affects the individual. They are inseparable from the point of view of addictions recovery. Everything must be in the healing process simultaneously."[1]

This story is from the Wellbriety Movement, which uses Native American experiences and traditions to support recovery and promote physical and spiritual wellness. The story is a mainstay in the recovery community and gives us guidance in creating recovery-friendly communities. In some communities, the poisons of anger, guilt, shame, and fear must be replaced by healing, hope, unity, and forgiveness to become a healthy place for everyone, including people in recovery and their families. While we usually think of recovery as something that the individual does, often with their family working on healing, the consequences of alcohol and drug use can harm entire communities. Over time, addiction weakens families and destroys neighborhoods, towns, and cities. The cycle—community conditions as a driver for addiction, which creates community decline, which in turn creates conditions for further addiction—is ongoing. Sick communities need recovery, too.[2]

A recovery-friendly community welcomes people in recovery with open arms, creates and maintains a stigma-free environment, actively builds recovery capital and recovery support services, and can help prevent further addiction and community decline. Regardless of your role or position—family member, neighbor, artist, person of faith, welder, business owner, librarian, law enforcement officer, doctor, lawyer, college dean, farmer, shipbuilder, carpenter, government official, and more—you can be part of creating and sustaining a recovery-friendly community where you live.

Public Health Strategies to Increase Recovery Capital

Local health departments and local coalitions are often the drivers for community-based interventions to promote health in a community. State and federal dollars often fund these interventions to address public health problems. In this sense, "community-based" means putting in place programs and policies to improve the health of individuals in a community defined by geographic boundaries and using community resources, like people and businesses, to accomplish specific health goals. Community-based interventions can also target broad health advances across the entire community or particular groups, for example, improving diabetes health outcomes in adults over fifty. "Community-based" also can mean that community organizations initiate changes and then draw on support from public health and health care professionals. In this way, families, schools, businesses, nonprofit organizations, and other groups in the community address their own problems, typically through some process of planning, action, and advocacy.[3] In reality, community-based interventions to address specific health issues like addiction are often some combination of these.

When it comes to recovery, community-based strategies can go a long way toward increasing recovery capital. Local communities—where we know each other and care for each other—can be nimbler in response to health problems than state or national organizations. This chapter provides examples of community-initiated projects using public health strategies to implement evidence-based interventions that increase recovery capital. In other words, this chapter has examples of the excellent work we can do in the community to encourage and support recovery for our family, friends, and neighbors.

Community Meetings

Holding town hall–style meetings is a meaningful, low-cost way to educate community members about addiction and recovery and link people in recovery to their neighbors. The purpose of such online or in-person meetings is to provide accurate information about addiction and recovery, highlight treatment and recovery resources in the area, and talk about specific ways people can get involved. Research shows that combining education with personal stories helps reduce stigma, so it's critical to include at least one person in recovery willing to tell their story and answer questions. Local doctors can provide accurate information about the disease of addiction, and substance use counselors can talk about local resources. If there's a recovery community center nearby, staff members can talk about opportunities for community members to get involved. After the presentations, it's essential to give people a chance to ask questions.

Many communities across the country have held town hall meetings like these, and people in attendance have felt the power of someone sharing their story of a life in addiction that ends in recovery. Such moments create empathy and hope for people who are struggling, their family members, and community members who despair at the levels of addiction and overdose deaths. For example, in one Maine town, a small local hospital held a series of meetings to talk about addiction and recovery to introduce its new treatment center. In another, a local church's Social Justice Committee hosted a series of community meetings on the root causes of addiction, the science of addiction, the importance of safe recovery housing, and the role of employment in recovery.

One good way to start a community meeting is to show the film *The Anon-ymous People*, a 2014 documentary that features some of the millions of Amer-icans living in recovery. It's available online for a minimal charge. Many other movies about addiction and recovery have been made in recent years, but I like *The Anonymous People* best because its sole focus is the good news of recovery. Many other movies include considerable dark content about people using drugs, which can be difficult and triggering for people in recovery who see it. For this reason, it's critical to preview movies with people in recovery before deciding which one to show a broad audience.

STEPS TO HOLDING A COMMUNITY LISTENING SESSION ABOUT RECOVERY

Faces and Voices of Recovery's *Community Listening Forum Toolkit: Taking Action to Support Recovery in Your Community* is a good place to start when you want to hold a community meeting. It's available at www .facesandvoicesofrecovery.org/blog/publication/community-listening -forum-toolkit. Boiled down to the essentials, these are the steps to a successful forum:

1. *Identify the Issue.* Possible topics include learning about community needs, informing the community about new recovery support ser-vices, or letting people know about current policy issues and how they can participate.

2. *Form a Planning Committee.* Be sure to include people in recovery.

3. *Decide on a Format.* Often, a community leader opens the meeting, followed by a person in recovery telling their story. The meeting continues with a knowledgeable speaker about the specific topic, a panel of people who reflect on the issue, and time for questions and answers.

4. *Select a Place and Date.* Be sure the location is convenient and sets the right tone for your meeting.

5. *Identify and Invite Speakers and Panelists.* Be sure to let them know what you want them to discuss and how much time they'll have. If possible, invite a respected community leader to kick off the forum.

6. *Prepare Materials to Distribute.* Handouts can include an agenda with the names, titles, and brief bios of presenters, FAQs on the topic, and fact sheets. In addition, participating organizations may have brochures and other information to share.

   Some reliable sources for fact sheets are:

   Faces and Voices of Recovery: www.facesandvoicesofrecovery.org

   Partnership to End Addiction: www.drugfree.org/drug-and -alcohol-news

   Drug Policy Alliance: www.drugpolicy.org

   National Institute on Drug Abuse: www.drugabuse.gov

7. *Invite and Register Attendees.* Putting up posters around town to promote the meeting is essential, but you may have more success reaching out to organizations and individuals directly via email and phone call invitations. Post messages and meeting invitations on social media. Be sure to send a reminder the day before the meeting.

8. *Promote the Forum.* Prepare a news release and share it, along with the meeting materials, with all local media. Partners that have public relations departments can help get the word out through their channels, too. Ask partners to promote the forum on their social media platforms.

9. *Hold the Forum.* Be sure to have a sign-up sheet so that you can contact attendees after the event. Have someone on hand to answer questions and take notes for follow-up. Some communities like to have a counselor available if sensitive topics come up that people want to talk about privately with a professional.

10. *Follow Up.* Make sure to follow up with everyone who attended, thanking them for their participation and inviting them to be part of the recovery community. This is a great way to recruit people to be part of recovery advocacy activities in your town and state.

Communication

Local newspapers, magazines, and TV stations are essential partners in communicating about addiction and recovery. Because reporters and broadcasters craft their news stories to capture the attention of busy readers and viewers, sometimes they use sensationalist language and images to draw them in. In the era of the opioid epidemic, images of needles, little packets of white powder (usually heroin or fentanyl), people in handcuffs, and people who have died from drug overdoses are common. Stories often open with descriptions of addicts whose lives fell apart. While these images and stories may sell newspapers or attract viewers, they are harmful to people in recovery. Some people find the images to be triggering and difficult to see. Others find language like "addict" offensive. Most people in recovery and their families want the additional message of healing and hope included in stories about addiction.

Community groups around the country have contacted local media to educate them about the potential harm of their stories and encourage them to use different words and images. For example, I was part of the Overdose Task Force in Portland, Maine. One of our strategies to reduce stigma was meeting in person with local reporters and news producers to give them concrete suggestions for positive stories about recovery and nonstigmatizing images and language. We started by creating a list of all local newspaper editors and reporters and radio and news stations' broadcasters. Then we identified the Associated Press's *AP Stylebook* entry for addiction.[4] One of our group drafted a letter to send to the editors, reporters, and broadcasters, thanking them for their coverage on addiction and suggesting they consider following the *AP Stylebook*. We added suggestions for recovery stories they could cover. We all weighed in on the letter, and then we emailed it along with a tip sheet and followed up with phone calls and in-person meetings when possible.

Our group had success with some newspapers and news outlets, and not others. One news anchor became a champion for recovery, identified himself publicly as a recovery ally, and included interviews with people in recovery in many of his stories about Maine's drug problems. Months later, when we noticed that articles and images were slipping back into the same stories of addiction as before, we realized that we had to return to this task every year or so.

SUGGESTIONS FOR THE MEDIA

In 2017, the Associated Press amended its *AP Stylebook* to reflect our changing understandings of substance use disorder:

- Use the medically precise and correct language, "substance use disorder," found in the *Diagnostic and Statistical Manual of Mental Disorders*, 5th edition *(DSM-5)*, rather than "dependence" or "addiction."

- Avoid words like "abuse" and "problem" in favor of the word "use" modified by "risky," "unhealthy," "excessive," or "heavy." "Misuse" is also acceptable.

- Separate the person from the disease and use person-first language, like "a person with substance use disorder" (or "opioid use disorder" or "alcohol use disorder") instead of "addict" or "alcoholic," except when used in a quotation or name of an organization.

- Avoid using the term "addicted babies." The correct medical term is "babies with neonatal abstinence syndrome."

Community Champion

One public health strategy for change is identifying leaders in the community who are "champions" for the cause. Recovery champions use their position and influence to change the conversation about addiction and recovery and bring resources to support recovery-friendly initiatives.

Bradford C. Paige, president and CEO of Kennebunk Savings, is a recovery champion. Kennebunk is the summer home of the George Bush family, and it's also home to Kennebunk Savings (KS), a community bank. KS was formed as a mutual institution, meaning the original founders didn't take an ownership interest or stock, but rather created the bank for the benefit of the community. KS remains mutual today, with no owners, but with a local board of directors that sets the strategic direction of the bank.

"For me, mutuality is all about patience," Brad says. "It's all about being patient and taking the long view with our three constituencies—our employees, our customers, and our communities. As a mutual institution, our communities are effectively our 'stockholders,' to which we pay 'dividends.' We give 10 percent of our annual earnings to local nonprofit organizations that help our communities thrive. We call it our Community Promise."

In 2019, Brad worked with the bank's leadership to shift their strategic financial goal from a target return on assets (profitability) to the Community Promise giveback. Now the strategic goal is to give back $1.5 million annually to the community. "Of course, this goal is tied to profitability in terms of the percentage of profits we need to get to that number, but it sends a better and more accurate message to the community about our priorities. Our reason to grow as an institution and expand into more communities is to support the community."

In 2016, KS started the Spotlight Fund. "Before that, we gave money to nonprofit organizations through the Community Promise program, but it was mostly reactive. We didn't have a plan," Brad explains. "In creating the Spotlight Fund, we wanted to proactively identify an issue affecting our communities, shine a light on it, and say, 'Hey, we're a bank, and we don't have anything to do with this issue, except we do, because we *all* do.'"

The Kennebunk Savings Community Relations team, which manages several programs and initiatives for KS, developed a planning process to identify areas of need in the community and then support organizations working to address those needs. "We looked for a very targeted, very local way to make a difference," Liz Torrance says. Liz is the bank's social responsibility manager and manages the Spotlight Fund; and she gets excited when she talks about the work the bank is doing. "We are part of this community," Liz says, "and as a mutual bank, being a socially responsible business is who we are. The bank's leadership knows that substance use is a big concern in the area, and they think of it as a 'we issue,' not a 'them issue.' Looking at the need for recovery support in the bank's service area, we asked the question, 'What can we do?'"

The bank turned to the recovery community, asking the best way to help create a recovery-friendly community. "We asked some pretty straightforward questions," Liz said, beginning with "Tell us about what you do and who you think we should talk to." As we went through that process things bubbled up, and it started to become clear what we could actually do on the local level to really help. First, the bank identified peer support programs based on research: recovery coaching, recovery community centers, and recovery residences. Through the Spotlight Fund, the bank then provided resources to existing nonprofits to support initiatives such as recovery coach trainings, planning for a recovery community center, and creating a training video for an association that supports recovery residences. The Spotlight Fund also supported transportation services, community trainings on adverse child-hood experiences, and prevention programming in schools. The bank wanted to share what it learned about substance use disorder. It held a conference with many of the subject matter experts they had come to know and invited area businesses to attend—challenging them to take action and offering themselves as a resource to get started. Finally, the bank "walked the talk" by becoming a designated Recovery Friendly Workplace.

KS leveraged its existing communications network and started a social media campaign to share what they'd learned about the effects of stigmatiz-ing language, adverse childhood experiences, and toxic stress. "We thought we could use our voice, not just to give money out, but also to be a resource and to educate the community. One of the biggest things that we know," Liz says, "is to never stop learning. We have to keep talking to people and learning more about what we can do. We also know it's OK to talk about recovery. The more you talk about it, the more you can help."

As a result of this planning, action, and advocacy in the community, KS has contributed more than $400,000 so far to community organizations to build recovery capital in the region in the form of stigma reduction, peer support, and increased access to treatment and recovery residences.

"Money is the easy part," Brad says. "Anybody can write a check or get a headline or take credit for a news story. But if you're really going to go at something like this proactively, you have to attack from all angles. So, yes, we gave quite a bit of money, but we have also addressed some ongoing needs."

Brad became a champion for recovery, speaking at events where people in recovery spoke. The meetings gave community members the chance to learn about substance use disorder and began building bridges between the recovery community and the broader community. "I can, as a mutual bank, do things that other corporate organizations are able to do, but at the end of the day, it comes down to your inner drive to make a difference. Go out and start the conversation about what to do about the substance use problem. You don't have to have money. If you're willing to be in a meeting, participate, give feedback. Everyone should be able to find an opportunity to do something they're passionate about. Figure out what the levers are in the community. In Kennebunk, it's the chamber of commerce and our chief of police. If you're already active, that's when you start getting your agenda into that organization," Brad says with passion. "Any place that you have that can create an outlet and additional conversation and action, figure out how to tap that."

Planning, Action, Advocacy

In 2016, the Metro Regional Coalition, a group of municipal leaders from seven cities and towns in Greater Portland, Maine, set out to accomplish the trifecta of public health work: planning, action, and advocacy. These are the classic steps to promote health and change health outcomes.

The Metro Regional Council, part of the larger Greater Portland Council of Governments (GPCOG) and consisting of city and town managers, school superintendents, police chiefs, recreation directors, and local government and school board members, had previously identified opioid use as the problem they wanted to address. They thought they might like to work on preventing youth from using opioids and supporting people in recovery, but they needed to know more about the issue. So, they sought and received funding from the regional public health council to engage in strategic planning and hold a leadership forum on the topic. They hired Liz Blackwell-Moore, a public health consultant who has devoted her career to substance use prevention and recovery, to help them. Her job was to educate the group, facilitate a regional assessment process to identify current efforts to address opioid misuse and gaps, and then support individual communities to create action plans and identify resources within the community to help complete the plans.

The first step was to understand what community leaders already knew and what towns were already doing to address opioid misuse. The consultant helped the Metro Regional Coalition survey people from fifty organizations to understand what was happening along the continuum from prevention to treatment to recovery in their communities in the region. Then the consultant led educational sessions that highlighted all that was already happening and the gaps in services. According to Liz Blackwell-Moore, "It was very important to show them that they are already addressing the problem in some ways. It helped them feel less hopeless and that there was something to build upon." The Metro Regional Coalition educational sessions also included learning about substance use disorder, its root causes, and evidence around preventing youth substance use and recovery support services. The consultant's presentations included the "public health parable" and information on adolescent brain development, trauma, and mental health issues as risk factors for initiating substance use and developing substance use disorder later in life. The presentations also included people in recovery telling their stories.

THE PUBLIC HEALTH PARABLE

(as told by the Communities Addressing Addiction & Opioid Misuse Project)

"There once was a town that had a waterfall. One day a group of towns-people are walking by the waterfall, and they notice people falling over the waterfall. They send a few people back to the town to get some nets, and they string up the nets to catch people as they are going over the water-fall. They quickly realize they aren't able to catch everyone as they are going over the waterfall. So, they send some people down to the lake below to pull people out of the lake. As they pull people out, they bring them back to the community to find support and healing. They realize, though, that there are still people deep in the waters that they are unable to save.

"Finally, they decide to send a group of people, including some people that were once in the river, to go upriver and figure out why people are falling in the river in the first place. They find a park at the edge of a cliff going into the river and people playing in the park, unaware of the cliff. So first, they put up a sign, letting people know of the cliff, then they put up a fence, and eventually, they try to move the park away from the cliff.

"This is where we find ourselves with the opioid problem. We are trying to stop people from dying by using naloxone and providing needle exchange. We are trying to support people to find treatment and recovery downriver, and we must also go upriver to stop addiction in the first place. But we can't stop any one of our efforts. We have to keep doing all of it to solve this problem."

"The connection between youth use of other substances and opioid use wasn't well understood," Liz Blackwell-Moore said. "Education about brain development, trauma, and mental health was critical. They didn't see how a kid who has a lot going for him but just smokes a lot of weed in high school can be the same young adult with opioid use disorder at age twenty-six."

ADOLESCENT BRAIN DEVELOPMENT

The human brain doesn't reach full maturity in young adults until the mid-twenties. Until then, the brain is "pruning" neural connections—clearing out what's not needed and building pathways for complex decision making. The adolescent brain appears to develop its emotional maturity before its cognitive abilities. The National Institute on Drug Abuse likens the adolescent brain to a car "with a fully functioning gas pedal (the reward system) but weak brakes (the prefrontal cortex). Teenagers are highly motivated to pursue pleasurable rewards and avoid pain, but their judgment and decision-making skills are still limited. This affects their ability to weigh risks accurately and make sound decisions, including decisions about using drugs."[5] Adolescents may apply the accelerator during periods of high emotion—such as in response to peer pressure, the thrill of taking risks, or the possibility of a short-term reward or positive outcome—without applying the brakes. The result may be risky decisions.

Adolescents may be prone to risky decision making when it comes to trying drugs or alcohol, a situation of high risk and high potential reward, especially if peers are present. Brain research suggests that early drug or alcohol use can negatively impact memory and learning. Brain development research also shows drug use during adolescence may increase the risk for developing a substance use disorder later in life. Among youth who began drinking when they were eleven to twelve years old, 7.2 percent had an alcohol use disorder within two years. For those who waited until age twenty-one to get drunk for the first time, 3.7 percent had an alcohol use disorder.[6]

Next, the public health consultant facilitated a leadership forum with seventy leaders from the Greater Portland area. After hearing about the root causes of addiction and evidence-based solutions, the Metro Regional Coalition chose to work together on stigma reduction and help each municipality decide what actions it wanted to take locally.

"The goal here isn't to just raise awareness about the problem. People already know what the problem is," Liz Blackwell-Moore explains. "Our fundamental goals are to move forward local leaders' understanding about the root causes of substance use disorders, and ultimately, especially, to increase their adoption and implementation of evidence-based strategies that we know are impactful and will reduce the opioid misuse problem."[7]

Falmouth, a wealthy suburb of Portland, was the first of the municipalities to complete the local process of assessment, leadership forum, and action plan development. First, municipal leaders formed a planning committee. Then, for the town assessment, school and municipal leaders answered questions on a template developed by the consultant to create a community scan of prevention, treatment, harm reduction, and recovery programs and initiatives already underway. The questions helped identify evidence-based work that was already occurring. Questions covered a range of topics—from "Does the school district have an assessment and referral process for students who violate the substance use policy?" to "Does your municipality have standards, guidelines, or policies in place for recovery residences?" (See Greater Portland Council of Governments, Communities Addressing Addiction and Opioid Misuse: A Project Toolkit for Cities and Towns, 2019, www.gpcog .org/282/Communities-Addressing-Addiction.)

Next, the planning committee used the results from the assessment to create a public dialogue of decision makers talking about the problem and possible solutions. After the public discussion, the planning committee created a strategic plan based on the assessment and gaps identified by community leaders. While the town had staff and resources to undertake the task, they also had some challenges. The planning committee got some pushback from residents who thought, "We don't have this problem" or "We're already doing enough."

The Falmouth planning committee hosted town meetings that included people in recovery telling their stories. The consultant made the same presentation that had been made to the GPCOG leaders (the public health parable, adolescent brain development, trauma, and mental health issues as risk factors for substance use disorder). The strategies the Falmouth planning committee selected were: to make recovery visible and reduce stigma by partnering with local organizations to host community meetings aimed at educating the community about prevention, recovery, and harm reduction; promote harm reduction by supporting naloxone trainings (naloxone is a medication that may reverse opioid overdoses) and explore the possibility of local needle disposal boxes; support parents by providing opportunities to learn about substance use disorder; implement a vaping intervention program in the high school; support educators and coaches with professional development opportunities, including restorative practices (focusing on repairing harm, taking responsibility, restoring relationships, and resolving conflict in place of punitive practices when wrongdoing occurs) instead of suspending students for violating school substance use policies; and create local standards for recovery residences. (See Appendix C for the "Falmouth Action Plan to Address Opioid Misuse.")

The Falmouth Town Council adopted the planning committee's action plan and began supporting it right away. In addition to professional development for educators, one concrete result was the police department hiring a recovery coach. The council's approval happened at the same time that a recovery residence opened in town to significant neighborhood opposition. This event presented the planning committee with an opportunity to talk to the community about supporting people in recovery. The town also participated in a regional workshop for town managers, town planners, and code enforcement officers on recovery residences, highlighting the role municipalities have in educating community members about the importance of recovery residences.

The town of Gorham also completed the process of assessment, community leader forums, and action plan development. In Gorham, municipal leaders felt like opioid misuse wasn't the primary issue. Instead, they were worried about addiction in general. So, the consultant broadened the process to meet their needs. This led to trainings of school administrators in using naloxone and more training of recreation department staff in positive youth development (programs, relationships, and environments that promote positive experiences for youth) and restorative practices. Liz Blackwell-Moore thinks engaging in the process also helped smooth out some of the concerns that town councilors had with a recovery residence that had recently opened. Some councilors had expressed reservations about having a recovery house right in town. However, after the forums, councilors expressed no outward resistance. "I can't say the change [in attitudes] was entirely 'caused' by the forums, but I think they helped," Liz Blackwell-Moore said.

In Portland, council members who came to the community leader forum told Liz Blackwell-Moore that they hadn't really thought about the implications of legal cannabis and early use of substances as it pertains to addiction to opioids or other drugs. Cannabis was legalized in Maine after a citizen referendum in 2016. Portland, as the largest municipality in Maine, potentially has the largest number of retail outlets. City councilors were in the midst of figuring out how many permits for legal cannabis retailers to give out, and at the time, they were talking about two hundred. The final policy allows for twenty-five legal cannabis retailers. Information about early substance use and adolescent brain development may have influenced their decision to cut the number of retailers considerably. According to Liz Blackwell-Moore, Portland is also revising school policies regarding substance use, moving to a more clinical approach to provide counseling to students who violate the policy instead of suspending them from school. In addition, the Portland Recreation Department staff received training in positive youth development, substance use prevention, and restorative practices for resolving conflict.

In 2019, after the three communities had gone through the assessment, community leader forums, and action plan development process, the Greater Portland Council of Governments published a toolkit for cities and towns to engage in this planning, action, and advocacy process. The toolkit is available free of charge at: www.gpcog.org/282/Communities -Addressing-Addiction.

SECTION 3
The Recovery Journey

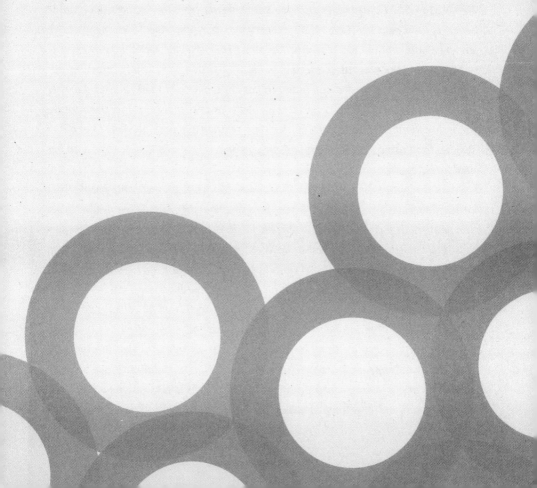

7

PATHWAYS OF RECOVERY

BRYN, A POISED, articulate attorney with a degree from the University of Maine School of Law, says her pathway to recovery was start-and-stop. "Some people have 'aha moments,' but not me," she says. "Entering recovery was a gradual process."

Bryn says she was raised by two loving, supportive parents who provided her with everything she needed and many things she wanted, but her childhood wasn't without difficulty. Bryn was warned in early adolescence that substance use disorder ran in her family and to be careful about her relationship with alcohol. That didn't stop her from using alcohol beginning early in high school as a way to cope with her need for acceptance and approval.

As a student at the University of Southern Maine, Bryn met some people from Portland's recovery community. When she asked how they knew they needed to get into recovery at such a young age—most were in their early twenties—all identified that "black hole feeling that had to be filled," which resonated with her and which she hadn't heard so accurately described until then. This led Bryn to think she might need to look at her relationship with alcohol. Still, the blackout drinking she frequently experienced was normalized by her other friends and by college culture, so she felt justified in continuing to drink often and to excess.

Bryn continued to drink off and on and began attending 12-step meetings for community and support. Her sobriety finally started while studying abroad in Spain during her junior year of college in spring 2013. She was lonely, having a hard time living abroad, and beginning to accept that her relationship with alcohol wasn't *healthy or "normal." She walked into an English-speaking 12-step meeting in Barcelona with almost no intention of getting sober. But that 12-step community simply felt right, familiar, and safe. Bryn has been in recovery since that day. Now she practices family law in Massachusetts.*

Bryn studied social justice issues as an undergraduate, then decided to pursue law. Her dedication to law school was potent, and she was able to channel the clear-headedness and passion that came with her sobriety. She (and others) spoke up about recovery throughout law school, and she served on a wellness task force that focused on substance use and mental health issues. One of the task force's accomplishments was making the law school's semi-annual gala more recovery friendly by creating a "no drinks" option for the event. Full-price tickets included two drinks; "no drinks" tickets were half price. This was one way for Bryn to make a difference in her profession. "The legal profession is drenched (pun intended) in alcohol and drugs," she says. "There is a national interest in addressing this."

Bryn was never homeless, didn't go to residential treatment, and always had reliable family support. She didn't have a severe substance use disorder (addiction); nevertheless, she had a problem with alcohol, considers herself in recovery, and was an active member of the campus recovery community. Her recovery journey was part of growing up and part of her self-exploration. "The whole point of recovery is to grow and blossom," Bryn says. Now she has moved away from attending 12-step meetings and has plugged into a "miraculous and supportive recovery community" in different states. She attributes this mainly to the relationships she made through her volunteer work with Young People in Recovery, a national advocacy organization. Her work, her community, and her relationships help her focus on a full life in recovery. "In so much of our culture, sobriety is synonymous with recovery, and recovery is synonymous with 12-step programs. I don't believe this to be true, although 12-step work is what worked for me in the beginning. A growing generation of people in recovery is open to different meanings of recovery and diverse pathways. I feel more fortunate than I can say to have found both human connection and purpose in my recovery, and I hope the same for everyone else, no matter their pathway into and through recovery."

Bryn's road to recovery wasn't straight, with the endpoint in view when she stopped drinking. Like many of us, she wasn't sure where she was going. She zigzagged on a path that included not drinking for a while, starting up again, and finally stopping altogether. She knew she couldn't grow and blossom on her own, and different people helped her along the way—counselors, professors, friends, family, and people she met in recovery circles.

This isn't unusual. Most people in recovery experiment with counseling, support groups, 12-step groups, spiritual and religious traditions, meditation, exercise, painting, poetry, personal coaches, recovery coaches, or any of hundreds of other services, support systems, and activities. Some people pursue abstinence-only recovery, others take medication for support, and others practice moderation in their alcohol and drug use.[1]

Pathways of Recovery

"Multiple pathways of recovery" is a phrase that people in the recovery field use to talk about the many different ways people sustain their recovery. (A "pathway *to* recovery" means how a person started in recovery.) Alcoholics Anonymous (AA) has been the mainstay of treatment and recovery in the United States, even though many people follow other pathways. Until recently, we didn't know much about those following different paths. Researchers at Harvard University conducted the National Recovery Survey to fill some of our knowledge gaps. The survey is the first national probability-based sample of US adults who self-identify as having resolved a significant alcohol or drug problem.[2] Of the people who identified as being in recovery, a little over half said their pathway was some form of "assisted recovery." This included formal treatment (residential or outpatient), group or individual counseling, detox services, medication, mutual aid organizations like AA, and community-based recovery support services like faith-based help, sober living, collegiate recovery centers, and recovery community centers—or some combination of those. The survey showed that, like Bryn, people typically draw on more than one type of support.

Natural Recovery
The National Recovery Survey found that most people who "used to have a problem with drugs or alcohol but no longer do" don't think of themselves as being in recovery. They are just living their lives without the problems caused by their drinking or drug use. Researchers call this natural recovery, spontaneous remission, or self-managed recovery, and call people who follow this

path self-remitters or self-healers. We don't know much about self-healers because they're hard to find. They don't show up in research on specific treatment modalities or mutual aid groups like 12-step programs because they recover without formal help. Studies from the 1990s show that about 80 percent of people who had a problem with alcohol but who are now in recovery are self-remitters. The figure is 71 percent for people who had used illegal drugs.[3]

For the most part, self-healers haven't used drugs or alcohol for prolonged periods. They generally have more recovery capital like financial stability, education, employment, and family support. Self-healers figured out on their own strategies that are similar to those taught in treatment models, like understanding the costs and benefits of using substances, avoiding the people, places, and things that are associated with using drugs or drinking, building meaningful relationships, creating a new social network with people who don't use, and finding meaningful things to do.[4] For younger adults, significant life changes like graduating from college or getting married were often keys to reducing or stopping their drug or alcohol use. Older adults began to see the consequences of their drinking or drug use before their lives entirely fell apart and decided to make a change. This doesn't mean they didn't have a problem or didn't work hard to create a better life. It just means alcohol or drugs didn't end up taking over their lives. *Recovery Allies* is about people with severe substance use disorder—addiction—which generally doesn't include self-healers.

Alcoholics Anonymous

For decades, AA has been the foundation for recovery in the United States. In fact, in some areas, AA has been the only game in town. For this reason, *Recovery Allies* devotes an entire chapter (chapter 8) to AA and other 12-step programs. In the United States, we use the 12-step vocabulary for talking about recovery because more often than not, people in 12-step programs have been the only people talking about recovery. People on other paths have just started to speak up. Until recently, there was no scientific evidence to support AA's effectiveness, even though physicians, pastors, counselors, and addiction clinicians have referred patients and clients to it for decades, and millions of people credit their sobriety to it. Now the evidence is in. Research shows that AA will provide a solid chance to help you with your drinking and improve your life.[5]

Medications for Addiction

The Food and Drug Administration has approved several prescription medications for the medical management of addiction. These are intended to be
used along with other recovery supports like counseling, recovery residences,
and peer support. They may be a stepping-stone to abstinence-based recovery for some people, and for others, they may be part of their lives for an
extended time. The most commonly prescribed medications are various formulations of buprenorphine (often referred to by the trade name Suboxone),
methadone, and naltrexone for treating opioid use disorder. Medications for
alcohol use disorder are disulfiram, acamprosate, and naltrexone. (See chapter 14, on Medications for Addiction.)

Specialty Treatment

For people who want or need professional help, finding the right treatment
at the right time can be challenging. The specialty care system for addiction
in the United States today is a jumble of community-based mental health
centers, hospitals, public and private counselors and residential treatment
centers, holistic healers, and charity care. Every state has a different way of
piecing together federal, state, and private funding, and every insurance company has various restrictions on what treatments they will pay for.[6] Many
facilities have long waiting lists. Add in dishonest tactics by some treatment
agencies to recruit patients,[7] and it's no wonder that people looking for help
get frustrated when trying to find the right treatment.

If you want to get the right treatment, a diagnosis is critical, but it's generally only people with a severe problem who receive a formal assessment and
diagnosis. About six out of ten people are self-healers who don't need specialty care. With a little support, they can self-correct. Another two of ten have
a moderate problem and might need professional help but not residential
treatment. With assistance, they can do well, too. Only about one or two in ten
people have a severe substance use disorder and need residential treatment.[8]

Sometimes, a person's problems with drugs and alcohol are apparent long
before they're ready to get help, and there's time for family members or friends
to see how severe the problem is and to look at different options. Other times,
a person is pretty good at hiding substance use until the situation spins out
of control. Either way, family members are left to figure out what to do. Most

families I talked with asked their family doctor for suggestions, confided in a trusted family member, friend, or pastor in hopes that that person would know how to find help, did countless internet searches, collected brochures from local treatment agencies, or sent away for information from expensive private residential facilities in country settings.

Karen and Eddie Walsh's story is typical. They have two children in recovery, their eldest daughter and their son. "We started the journey with our daughter twelve years ago. Neither of our families had any experience with addiction, and at that time, neither did our friends. We didn't have a lot of people to turn to, and there were not a lot of resources out there," says Karen. "That's one of the things we found to be most difficult. There were counselors, but we ended up trying to reach out to other people, desperate for some advice for how we should be handling the situation."

Karen and Eddie found a support group for family members of people in active addiction and recovery, and that made all the difference. "As parents, we were lonely, depressed, angry," Eddie explains. "When we talked to other parents who had the same problem and people in recovery, we started to feel hope. We really didn't know recovery existed, and we needed to learn.

"We learned from other parents and people in recovery to offer help to our daughter and provide her help when she was ready for it, to tell her we're willing to be there for her but not to give her money or to provide things that she would misuse."

Karen continues, "As parents, we always think we have to fix things. We have to make this right. I can remember researching and printing articles and leaving them on my daughter's bed, thinking she would find them helpful because I found them helpful, and that would make a difference. We finally realized that change is not going to come from us; it's going to come from her. You can't fix it; they have to fix it."

Karen and Eddie's main message to parents is "When your kids ask for help, you need to be there. You need to do whatever you can do when she says, 'I'm ready. I need to go someplace for help.'"

Detox and Medically Supervised Withdrawal

"Detox" is short for detoxification and refers to the period immediately after stopping drug or alcohol use, when the body clears substances. Depending on the substance, this can be potentially life-threatening and require hospitalization (alcohol), physically excruciating (opioids), or psychologically and physically painful (most substances). For people with severe substance use disorder, a typical course is to detox at home, in jail, in the hospital, or in a specialized detox center where it is referred to as medically supervised withdrawal. Medically supervised withdrawal takes place under the care of medical and mental health professionals who manage severe symptoms and possible medical complications of withdrawal. Social detox takes place in nonmedical settings, usually with social workers and peers providing comfort and support. People without access to either of these facilities detox at home, alone, or with friends or family. Most jails give no support for people who detox there.

Some people just want to detox on their own and may not understand the risks of doing that without support and follow-up. Going through detox—whether in a medical or social detox center or somewhere else—doesn't mean a person is past their addiction, that the work is done. Detox only leads the body and mind toward healing, *but it doesn't usually result in sustained recovery without recovery supports.*

Treatment

Residential treatment is what most people think of when they say "treatment" or "rehab," and many people have benefited from it. Most treatment facilities follow some version of the Minnesota Model, developed by the Hazelden Foundation—a renowned nonprofit treatment provider—in the 1940s. The model is based on abstinence and the cornerstone that "alcoholics and addicts can help each other." People are inpatients for twenty-eight days and are expected to behave responsibly, attend lectures on the 12 steps of Alcoholics Anonymous, attend to the details of daily life, tell their stories, and listen to each other. The aim is to help patients shift from a "life of isolation to a life of dialogue." Professionals provide counseling and medical care as needed, and nonprofessional staff in recovery provide peer support. Each patient works with staff to develop an individualized treatment plan. When possible, active family involvement is part of the program, and staff provide education for them, too. Suboxone may be added as adjunct medical care for people with opioid use disorder.[9]

There's no evidence that twenty-eight days is the optimal number required for sustained recovery. The twenty-eight-day stint is based on insurance company reimbursement requirements rather than science and has become the industry standard. Some residential treatment facilities offer services that aren't evidence-based, and some charge exorbitant amounts, with promises of "90 percent success rates." It's worth checking around to be sure that what the facility provides is based on science and research. Consulting the National Institute on Drug Abuse's *Principles of Drug Addiction Treatment: A Research-Based Guide,* 3rd edition, is one good way to do this.[10] Some people benefit from standard residential treatment, and others don't.[11] Nearly everyone benefits from recovery support services long after they've left treatment.

Sometimes people go willingly to treatment and self-refer after a "wake-up call" of being thrown out of the house or arrested or having a religious or spiritual experience. Family members may stage an intervention—a meeting where family members tell the person who is in active addiction about the negative impact their use is having—as a way to create an opening for the person to accept residential treatment. (Evidence is mixed that family interventions, like those seen on the A&E network's show *Intervention,* effectively get loved ones to engage in treatment. Family members should seek a mental health professional's assistance to facilitate an intervention of this kind to be sure the intervention is done safely.) Sometimes treatment is court-ordered. Judges may order some form of treatment due to an offense such as driving under the influence or a drug-related crime.

Faith and Spirituality

At some point in their recoveries, some people find great comfort and support in their faith and return to the faith community of their childhood or find a new and welcoming congregation. Some people have a religious conversion that brings them out of addiction and closer to God. Still others appreciate the support that faith-based residential treatment and other programs provide.[12]

Holistic Healing and the Arts

Mind-body practices like yoga and meditation that create mindfulness are common paths of healing in recovery.[13] Yoga practices that are trauma-informed or incorporate the 12 steps are also popular. Some people find that artistic expression like writing, painting, or singing helps their recovery.

Other Pathways

AA is the most well-known mutual aid organization, but there are many other peer support programs and fellowships, including:

- The Wellbriety Movement and White Bison are culturally based healing programs for Native Americans and others who wish to participate.

- Refuge Recovery is based on the Buddhist practices of meditation.

- SMART (Self-Management and Recovery Training) is a science-based, peer-led program based on cognitive behavioral therapy.

- LifeRing Secular Recovery is an abstinence-based program that helps individuals build personal recovery plans and receive peer support.

- Women for Sobriety is an abstinence-based mutual aid program for women that focuses on building self-esteem and emphasizes recovery as the individual's accomplishment.

- Secular Organizations for Sobriety is a network of independent abstinence-based support groups that aren't religious or spiritual in nature.

- Moderation Management is a program of peer-led local groups for people concerned about their drinking and who want to make positive changes in the amount or the way they drink.

- Celebrate Recovery is a Christian program based on scripture and the 12 steps of Alcoholics Anonymous.

- Phoenix Multisport is a physical activity program that offers climbing, hiking, running, strength training, yoga, cycling, and other activities for people in recovery.

Will They Recover?

Family members want to know, "Will my loved one recover?" And the answer is "probably." The most likely outcome of substance use disorder is recovery. The National Survey on Drug Use and Health, conducted annually by the Substance Abuse and Mental Health Services Administration, shows that 75 percent of people with a problem with substances (mild, moderate, or severe) recovered.[14] Of those who have a severe problem and participate in professional treatment, about 50 percent recover.[15]

Treatment is an essential gateway to recovery for some people. Our stereotype of the "revolving door" of treatment for people with substance use problems and the associated belief that "treatment doesn't work" aren't based on fact. Results from the National Recovery Survey showed that most people resolved their alcohol or drug problem with one or two serious attempts. For people with the most severe issues, it took an average of five tries. For context, the number of quit attempts for people who smoke cigarettes is between six and thirty.[16]

A Powerful, Controversial Statement

"You're in recovery when you say you are" may be the most controversial statement in the recovery community. And it's perhaps the most powerful. Historically, being in recovery has meant being abstinent. Now, with medications for addiction, new understandings of recovery as a process of change toward wellness, and changing attitudes toward moderate drug use, a culture war has developed between those who insist on abstinence and those who find other paths. Declaring "you're in recovery when you say you are" in a group of people in recovery usually results in an animated discussion that highlights divisive either/or thinking, with "true recovery is abstinence" on one side and "recovery includes pathways with medications for addiction, psychedelics, or recreational use of other substances" on the other side. The statement also stirs discussions about making the boundaries of recovery so broad that a shared identity no longer exists. This gets at the core of "What is recovery?"

An "abstinence-only" pathway through Alcoholics Anonymous has helped millions of people, and many of them are passionate about that. People in the 12-step community (including people who participate in Narcotics Anonymous, Cocaine Anonymous, and others) draw strength and inspiration from the 12 steps and the fellowship of meetings with fellow people in recovery. For them, this approach creates hope for people in dark places when they're in active use, and it lays out a road map to wellness. Complete abstinence is a critical part of their recovery.

As an organization, AA has no opinion on medications for addiction (or on any other pathways, for that matter), and meetings are open to people using psychiatric medications, including medications for addiction. Still, enough people in AA believe that those medications simply "replace one drug with another" and that a stigma exists for people taking them. From this perspective, people recovering from opioid use disorder who are on Suboxone or methadone are "not really in recovery"; and that the same is true of people who take a harm reduction approach and use cannabis or entheogen (psychedelic) substances as part of their recovery. Within some AA groups, a pecking order of recovery has resulted, where the "best" recovery is abstinence-based, followed by taking medications for addiction, followed by moderate use and harm reduction.

Now a new generation of people doubts the value of being anonymous or abstinent, and they're looking at recovery more broadly. People in their twenties and thirties have seen more pathways, like medications for addiction and harm reduction, finding acceptance. They have a more open attitude toward different paths of recovery, and this is spreading to some older people in long-term recovery.

When all is said and done, the best recovery path is the one that a person chooses that moves them toward health and wellness. Accepting another person's path is just as important within the recovery community as in the broader community. We may want something different for the people in our lives who are in recovery—a different job, a different partner, a different way of living. But even if we disagree with the path our loved one has taken, we do a better job at supporting their recovery when we respect their chosen journey.

Honesty Liller, who has been in recovery for fifteen years and runs a recovery community organization in Richmond, Virginia, summed it up well when she said, "What's your path, bro? What do you want in your personal recovery? I just wish people would just shut the hell up and respect each other's recovery."

What Can Allies Do?

For Family Members and Friends

- Ask your family member or loved one open-ended questions about their recovery journey to learn more about it. If they go to support groups, what do they find most helpful? If they interact with peers, what do they like about that? Ask them the best way for you to support their journey, and be prepared to step up and do what they ask. If they're reluctant to talk about it, respect their personal boundaries and the requirement of anonymity of 12-step programs.

- Be sure to take care of yourself! When a family member enters recovery, the family dynamics can change a lot. Think about your own physical and emotional needs, and seek out support. Some people benefit from help from their church community or clergy. Others prefer secular support groups. Al-Anon is a mutual aid group for adults who have been affected by someone else's drinking or who grew up with someone who drank and were affected by that. Alateen is for teens who are affected by someone else's drinking. Some communities have local support groups for family members. Check your local recovery community center for what's available in your area.

- If your friend or family member attends Alcoholics Anonymous or another type of support group, ask if it would be OK for you to participate with them. Many groups are open to people who aren't in recovery, and attending is a great way to learn and get to know people in your loved one's circle of peers. Most people who aren't in recovery walk away from their first meeting with an appreciation for the work that goes into getting well and more compassion for people in recovery.

- Residential treatment and 12-step programs aren't for everybody, but sometimes they are the only item on the menu. If your friend or family member isn't finding AA helpful or didn't like being in rehab, ask if they're open to your help in finding other pathways, including online options.

- Unless you're in recovery yourself, resist the temptation to suggest what you think would be a better way. Recovery is a self-directed journey, and peers in recovery are often more helpful than family members with suggestions. Family members can help by being caring and non-judgmental with minimal suggestions.

- Family members who are interested in a family intervention should seek the assistance of a mental health professional. Even though it may feel good to "finally be doing something," the evidence is mixed about the success of this type of intervention.

For Social Workers and Health Care Providers

- Look at the recovery pathways in this chapter and make sure you are familiar with each one. Take a look at your patient panel or client base and be sure you know which pathway(s) each person follows. If you don't know, find a way to ask as part of their regular appointment.

- Check out what's in your community. Where do people go to detox? Where are the residential treatment facilities nearby? What types of counseling are available? Where and when are the AA meetings? Where are other support groups? Where are the Suboxone prescribers and methadone clinics? Where are the recovery community centers? Which organizations engage peer support (recovery coaches)?

- Develop a referral protocol that starts with asking the patient what would support their recovery, and help connect them with resources.

- Use your voice to publicly support all pathways to recovery and show up for community meetings and recovery events like rallies or walks.

For Clergy and Faith Leaders

- Spend some time learning about addiction and about how your faith understands it. If you know people in your congregation who are in recovery, reach out to them privately and ask how you can support their path.

- Offer public statements that make it clear your congregation welcomes people on all paths of recovery, and back them up by showing up at recovery events in your town, such as community meetings or recovery rallies.

For Holistic Healers

- Learn about recovery and how your healing art can contribute to wellness for people in recovery and offer, for example, recovery-friendly yoga classes.

For Artists

- Learn about recovery and how your art can contribute to wellness for people in recovery. Consider holding writing workshops for people in recovery and their families or recovery poetry readings or recovery rap competitions. Look into hosting a recovery art show or including works by artists in recovery at local galleries.

8

ALCOHOLICS ANONYMOUS
AND 12-STEP PROGRAMS[1]

IN 1992, OLIVIA was in crisis. Although she'd been homeless before, now she had an apartment and thought things were finally going to get better. But she couldn't stop drinking.

Her drinking and drug use were out of control, and she no longer had people she could turn to for help. She had blown up every single bridge to others. "I was twenty-four years old, and at that time in my life, I felt so disconnected from the human race," she explained. "My life had gotten very small—a biker bar, a convenience store for cigarettes and what little food I was eating, and my apartment, which was gross. So that was my life. My world was really small, and humans scared me."

After a visit from state authorities concerned about her children's well-being, Olivia drank again, and the following day she called a statewide crisis helpline. An operator connected her with a member of Alcoholics Anonymous (AA). A woman named Shirley picked her up and took her and her children to an AA meeting. Olivia was drunk when she walked into the meeting, but she remembers that "everyone was so happy, it was bright and sunny and there was a lot of laughter, and you could feel this great energy in the room. An older man was holding a baby, and there were forty-five to fifty people. It was thirty years ago, and I remember it like it was yesterday."

At the meeting, Olivia sat quietly for the entire hour. Shirley arranged for Olivia to be picked up and taken to another AA meeting in the evening. When the time came, Olivia went to the biker bar instead.

Olivia kept being drawn back to AA, even while she continued drinking. She showed up drunk to meetings for a while before she finally quit. Mostly, she showed up at a social club in town with space for socializing, coffee, food, and meetings for people in recovery. Bill, who had attended AA for years, was there most of the time and told her, "Just keep coming back," and she did. Bill and others looked out for her and connected her with women who made sure she got home safely after meetings. "For years after, once I was sober, I'd see Bill at a meeting, and he'd look at me and shake his head and say, 'Miracle!' and he meant me!"

Months later, her life spun entirely out of control. Once again, state officials stepped in, sent her to rehab, and temporarily removed her children from her apartment. After leaving rehab and drinking again, her children were permanently removed and placed in the custody of family members. "I went to a halfway house and spent six months learning to live. During rehab, I learned that I really am an alcoholic. But after rehab, when I tried to control it and found that I couldn't, I knew I was in trouble. I proved again and again that once I started, I couldn't stop. I honestly didn't think I had a problem with alcohol. I thought my problem was blacking out. If I could only figure out how to drink without blacking out, everything would be OK!" she said with a laugh.

"The halfway house gave me a safe, secure place to land, gave me structure, counselors to talk to, and a group of people that were doing what I was doing— learning to live without drugs or alcohol," Olivia explained. One of the requirements of the houses, like many recovery residences, was to go to AA meetings. "I resented that because I was a busy woman! Oh, sure, I was a busy woman with no job, no kids, and one chore a week to do at the house, and my attitude was 'How dare you tell me what to do!'" Olivia chuckled as she told me this part of her story, and then she got serious. "I got heavily involved in AA, and it saved my life and changed the lives of my children.

"People in AA knew what I needed way before I knew," Olivia said. "They knew I needed a home group, a commitment, and a sense of responsibility so that I would feel included. A home group is made up of members who work together to keep the meeting going. You make a commitment to show up once a week, you vote on aspects of the meeting, and you have a position in that home group—greeter, chip person,

secretary, treasurer, floor sweeper—every position is important because it keeps the meeting going. You have a purpose, and the people in your home group become your family—your sister or your grandfather or the family you never had. At first, I cleaned the ashtrays. Then I was a greeter, and then I put the chairs away after the meeting. I had to show up every week at that meeting because I had that job to do. I needed to help keep the meeting running, and that responsibility helped me feel like I was giving something back to the group of people that put on the meeting.

"The people in AA also knew I needed a sponsor, somebody to guide me around 'the halls and the steps.' I started to learn that I didn't have to do anything alone anymore. Sponsors shared their own experiences with the program. They were women who had been where I had been, hopeless and full of despair, but weren't there now and felt free and serene. A sponsor shared what worked for her and walked me through the steps, which helped me see that something had the power to keep me away from drinking. I certainly had proved to myself that I didn't have that power.

"My sponsor and I started building a relationship with a simple, basic structure, which is so important in those early weeks and months. She had me call her every day, read from AA's Daily Reflections *every morning, and tell her my plan for the day. As I started doing those readings, I started to read things that I felt emotionally but couldn't verbalize. When I read it, I thought, 'Yes, yes, that's what I'm feeling!' and that meant somebody else felt it, too, and I wasn't alone. I started to feel connected with the larger picture of what Alcoholics Anonymous is.*

"I learned from the other women in AA," Olivia said. "Women traveled in packs, and we did everything together. We went to meetings, and we went out for coffee or lunch. We protected our own. There were women ahead of you and women behind you, and you didn't go to a meeting alone. We went on commitments together. [A commitment is when home group members go to other meetings together to share their experience, strength, and hope.] We said what our lives were like, what happened to change that, and what our lives are like now so that we could inspire more people, especially other women.

"It's so important for people to understand that AA isn't just a program; it's a way of life. It's a framework to live life, not just not to drink. AA isn't about not drinking; it's about learning how to live. Oddly enough, it really works best when I pass along to other women what worked for me."

Most people have heard of Alcoholics Anonymous (AA), and many think it's synonymous with recovery. That's probably because AA is the most common place people look for help for their alcohol problems, and it forms the foundation of treatment and recovery in the United States. AA is part of most residential treatment programs, and the treatment workforce is made up primarily of people in recovery whose path includes AA. Many of the concepts and phrases we hear about addiction and recovery like "hitting rock bottom" and "once an alcoholic, always an alcoholic" come from the program.

AA is an anonymous and peer-led program made up of thousands of meetings every day around the world. Each AA meeting is autonomous, and members determine the focus of their meetings. As a result, some meetings will be a better fit than others for any one person. For example, some focus on reading "The Big Book," written by the founders of AA, and others focus on current meditation practices. Because it's free and easily accessible, mental health counselors, law enforcement, judges, and health care providers often refer clients to local meetings to support their recovery. No referral is necessary, though. Meetings are welcoming, and membership is open to anyone with a desire to stop drinking, so many people simply show up at a meeting looking for support. Some meetings are designated for beginners. Some are open to loved ones and people who want to learn, and others are for AA members only.

AA is a mutual help organization that started in 1935 for people with alcohol use disorder. While it is associated with early Christian movements, AA has no religious or political affiliation. It was designed around the "12 steps." Other mutual help programs like Narcotics Anonymous (founded in 1953), Gamblers Anonymous (founded in 1957), Overeaters Anonymous (founded in 1960), and Cocaine Anonymous (founded in 1982) are based on the same 12 steps. Each program, however, has its own history and culture. All programs promote an abstinence-based path to sobriety, to a "spiritual transformation of personal identity within which alcohol [or drugs] no longer has a place."[2] AA views the nature of alcohol use disorder as an incurable and fatal disease, as an illness that only a spiritual experience can conquer. The only way to stop the progression of the disease is to stop drinking altogether, surrender to a higher power, and then rebuild a new identity and a new life through a daily program of spiritual practice. Doing this will result in a life full of richness and blessings beyond what was possible during active drinking.

AA is an essential path of recovery for many, many people. It is a map to a contented life in recovery for people with severe alcohol use disorder and helps forge their new identity in recovery. The program helps thousands by providing guidance, feelings of belonging and hope, and a community where people learn to socialize without drugs or alcohol. Sharing life stories is at the heart of AA. Members tell, retell, and refine their own stories of "who I was before I became an alcoholic, who and what I became through the progression of my alcoholism, and how my life has changed as a result of AA." Newcomers can see themselves in the stories of dark emotions, dishonest behaviors, and failed attempts to stop drinking through willpower alone and feel hope when they see how others have turned their lives around. Telling—and retelling—one's own story can serve as a reminder of the importance of sobriety and can inspire others. AA meetings create opportunities to connect and reconnect with people with similar experiences. The experiences, strength, and hope shared at meetings can be lifesaving.

In addition to personal stories, a daily "centering ritual," like reflecting on one's conduct or meditating, helps members put their recovery first, every day. AA slogans like "Easy Does It," "This Too Shall Pass," "One Day at a Time," and "Keep It Simple" are shorthand self-talk that can help people stay focused on their recovery when difficult emotions creep in and create the desire to drink. Acts of personal responsibility like making the bed every morning and maintaining good hygiene and eating habits, and acts of service like supporting another person's recovery or volunteering in the community, are also essential parts of building a new identity and life.

Many AA members say they benefit from the spiritual focus of AA and point to their own "spiritual awakening" as evidence. This awakening usually isn't a single revelation, but rather the result of the journey from the pain of addiction to admitting failings (steps 4 and 5), character reconstruction (steps 6 and 7), rebuilding personal relationships, and in so doing, rebuilding identity (steps 8, 9, and 10), seeking redemption (step 11), and gaining gratitude from a complete understanding of one's limitations and ability to help others because of those limitations (step 12). It is the gratitude and helping others that leads to a profoundly satisfied spirit, and this is the "spiritual awakening" that members usually refer to.

ALCOHOLICS ANONYMOUS: THE 12 STEPS[3]

1. We admitted we were powerless over alcohol—that our lives had become unmanageable.

2. Came to believe that a Power greater than ourselves could restore us to sanity.

3. Made a decision to turn our will and our lives over to the care of God as we understood Him.

4. Made a searching and fearless moral inventory of ourselves.

5. Admitted to God, to ourselves, and to another human being the exact nature of our wrongs.

6. Were entirely ready to have God remove all these defects of character.

7. Humbly asked Him to remove our shortcomings.

8. Made a list of all persons we had harmed and became willing to make amends to them all.

9. Made direct amends to such people wherever possible, except when to do so would injure them or others.

10. Continued to take personal inventory and when we were wrong promptly admitted it.

11. Sought through prayer and meditation to improve our conscious contact with God, as we understood Him, praying only for knowledge of His will for us and the power to carry that out.

12. Having had a spiritual awakening as the result of these Steps, we tried to carry this message to alcoholics and to practice these principles in all our affairs.

"Some people think that addicts and alcoholics drink and drug to escape their problems. I don't believe that," says John, a sixty-year-old man. "I believe addicts and alcoholics drink and drug not because they are 'running from,' but rather because *they are 'searching for.' In my case, my search had become more desperate as every-thing else had failed, and I began putting anything that altered my emotional state into my body. Which drug worked best? How much did I need? There was never any concern for danger. After I'd been using a while, it was no longer about 'getting high'; it was about not being sick, trying to function in a job, or looking mostly normal to family and friends."* John experienced seizures, car crashes, overdoses, blood infec-tions, and federal prison, and nothing deterred him from using drugs.

John explained that it was his own attitudes and beliefs that prevented him from objectively seeing himself. He wasn't able to see how he had grown thin and gaunt, with dull eyes. *"There was no recognition of the repeated behaviors of waking up, feeling sick, scheming to acquire more drugs or alcohol, using, crashing, and repeat,"* John says. *"Denial was firmly entrenched in my psyche, and there was little my family and friends could do to smash through to the old 'me' buried underneath.*

"Miracles do happen," John went on, *"and finally, the repeated pain and suffering made me teachable. For a person who had always controlled the outcome and could expect success with hard work and diligence, it was a difficult lesson to hear that my problem wasn't lack of power but rather that I was powerless over my addiction. It was only by accepting the idea, at a cellular level, that no amount of wishing, planning, hoping, or willpower would allow me to control my use of alcohol and drugs. The idea that my body and brain react differently when these chemicals are put into my body gradually became a central notion I needed to accept or perish.*

"I gave 12-step meetings a try. By attending meetings and hearing other people's stories, I began to identify with the others in the group. I heard what they did, how out of control their lives had become, and the steps they took to get better. I wanted the heal-ing and peace they had experienced. I wanted what they had, and I became willing.

"At one of the first meetings I attended, an old-timer said to me, 'Hey, this is really easy. All you need to do is change two things.' I eagerly awaited as he paused, looked at me wryly, and said, 'You just have to change your attitudes and behaviors.' It took a minute, but it sunk in—I would have to change everything."

Research and the 12 Steps

The National Recovery Survey conducted by researchers at Harvard found that about 25 percent of people who identified as being in recovery partic-ipated in some mutual help organization, including AA. Most people who aren't self-healers pursue more than one recovery type of assistance, so AA is one of several supports, such as formal treatment, medication, counseling, and community-based recovery support services like recovery coaches.[4]

A recent systematic literature review by researchers Drs. John Kelly, Keith Humphreys, and Marica Ferri found strong scientific evidence to support AA's effectiveness in helping people recover from alcohol use disorder.[5] Research on Narcotics Anonymous shows similar results for people with opioid use disorder,[6] including those who are taking medications for addiction.[7] The review of AA literature found that people who participate in AA are 20–60 percent more likely to end up abstinent than people who don't; that AA is as good as or better in supporting abstinence and reducing drinking than meditation, education, cognitive behavioral therapy, or outpatient treatment provided by doctors or social workers; and that AA is also as good or better at reducing the consequences of alcohol use, such as strained relationships and problems at work. An earlier study by Dr. John Kelly and others arrived at a similar conclusion and added that AA's effectiveness might not be due to content explicitly related to spirituality and alcohol, but instead to the fact that it is free with easy access at any point in the recovery journey, and participants can "dose" themselves according to their needs.[8]

In short, AA can help people get sober, stay sober, drink less, and suffer fewer consequences of drinking.

AA saves money, too, by reducing health care and law enforcement costs and lost productivity at work. For people with few resources and no access to mental health or treatment services, AA meetings in churches and community centers are free, accessible safe havens when they have no place else to go.

AA works differently for different people. For most, it helps by changing social networks—dropping drinkers and adding people who don't drink. It helps by having a sponsor, who is like a mentor or advisor, who coaches people through the early weeks and months of recovery and any other time. Other members in the program inspire hope by the lives they lead. AA also works by demonstrating skills to new members about staying sober, coping with difficult situations, thinking differently about themselves, increasing self-confidence, reducing cravings and impulsivity, and maintaining motivation for abstinence.

For some people, being in a supportive community is the most important part of AA. Others stay well by helping others—step 12 admonishes members to "carry this message to alcoholics"—which is a significant component of many members' recovery paths. Evidence shows that helping others is good for our health generally, and AA provides its members with countless opportunities to "give back."[9]

Many AA members say the spiritual focus of AA is central to maintaining their recovery. To date, there is no solid research to support or refute this. A common misperception is that members must believe in God to get well, which isn't the case. The evidence shows that atheists or agnostics who attend AA share the same benefits of AA as religious people (but they are less likely to seek help through AA).[10]

What Can Allies Do?

For Everyone

- Learn about 12-step programs and find them in your community. Each 12-step program has a wealth of free information online about "the steps" and recommended meeting formats. They also have information online about where meetings are held and links to free mobile apps to locate meetings. Local recovery community centers also keep lists of meeting locations and times. The most common 12-step meetings are Alcoholics Anonymous, Cocaine Anonymous, Crystal Meth Anonymous, Narcotics Anonymous, and Marijuana Anonymous. AA meetings are by far the most common. Many people with addictions to substances other than alcohol attend AA meetings.

- Check out a 12-step meeting by going to the AA meeting guide at the Alcoholics Anonymous website: https://alcoholicsanonymous .com/find-a-meeting/. Some AA meetings are open to the public. These tend to be "speaker meetings," sometimes a celebration of the time in sobriety of a member, who will tell their story. The format of speaker meetings is always the same: what life was like during active use, what happened when it changed, and what life is like today.

- Ask your loved one or friend with children if they would like you to babysit while they go to meetings. For single parents with young children, going to a 12-step meeting regularly can be challenging. Most meetings don't provide childcare, and while some meetings are happy to have children attend, parents may want to experience the support of the meeting without their children present. Friends, neighbors, and family members can help by offering to babysit at the same time each week, to make regular meeting attendance possible.

For Community Organizations

- Reach out to 12-step groups when you're looking for volunteers. Among people in any stage of recovery, but especially early recovery, "giving back" is an integral part of healing. Ask what types of volunteer tasks people in recovery might like. For example, humane societies can find dog walkers; clothing closets can find people to help sort and price used clothing; food pantries can find people to help lift boxes, fill shelves, and serve meals. The list goes on and on.

9

RECOVERY AND STIGMA

IN MAY 2015, I attended the third annual Maine Harm Reduction Conference and met David, a burly, athletic man in his mid-thirties. He was a caseworker at Preble Street, a bustling resource center for men, women, and children who live in homeless shelters or on the streets of Portland, Maine. He'd been out of prison and in recovery from addiction for four years and was an outspoken advocate for recovery support services. David was in a social work program at the University of Southern Maine and was looking forward to graduating the following spring. At the conference, held in basement meeting rooms of Portland Public Library, he agreed to fill in for someone who hadn't shown up. Sitting alone in a white plastic chair in front of about fifty people, he talked about stigma and shame and how the language we use to talk about addiction and recovery really matters. David hadn't prepared any notes, and yet he was incredibly articulate.

I will never forget what he said because it was heart-stopping in its raw honesty. He said, "When you call me an addict, you take away everything that is lovely about me."

In November, just six months later, he died from a drug overdose. His family and the recovery community were devastated. He had been a role model and inspiration for so many people. In the basement of Preble Street Resource Center, his memorial service was a tribute to his dedication to helping people and making sure they were treated with dignity and respect. Tragically, David's friends think he was too ashamed of his renewed alcohol and heroin use to ask for help, a victim of the same stigma he had talked about at the conference.

Stigma happens when we shun people who don't conform to our social norms. As a community, we view people who use drugs, people with alcohol problems, and people in recovery as losers. With verbal and nonverbal cues, we let them know they don't measure up and don't belong. We feel justified in condemning their behavior. Stigma reinforces our social norms by separating "us" from "them."

Stigma divides us as a community rather than unites us, making it even harder for people in recovery to have respect for themselves. Reducing stigma is one of the most critical challenges community members can take on. We can all do something to lessen stigma, and every person in recovery I've spoken with says it can make a huge difference in their lives. Shame and silence, they tell me, make recovery more difficult.

Addiction is one of the most stigmatized human conditions, and people around the world, from every culture, experience shame associated with their addictions.[1] This stigma carries into recovery. "Once an alcoholic, always an alcoholic" is a saying from Alcoholics Anonymous that has seeped into our cultural understanding of addiction. The saying (and by extension, "once an addict, always an addict") is used in much of the treatment world and means that once people with severe alcohol use disorder begin to drink compulsively, they can never go back to social or "normal" drinking. The only healthy way forward is abstinence. While this is true for some people, it can feel like a life sentence of shame for others.

We all have a past, and most of us aren't proud of every single aspect of it. We prefer to focus on the positive things in the past or the great things we're doing in the present and our hopes for the future. If we do the same for people in recovery, we make room for their hopes, too. This can be hard, especially if the actions of those we love when they were in active addiction embarrassed or wounded us. We may be angry, resentful, or ashamed, but we deliver much-needed compassion to people working on getting well and staying healthy when we focus on hope.

Stigma and the Opioid Crisis

The stigma around addiction has long been a part of American culture. It varies considerably from one community to the next, so it's hard to generalize.

Young people may have different attitudes than their parents or grandparents, just as people who have used drugs themselves may have different outlooks than those who haven't. Feelings vary from one ethnic group to another and from one religious group to another as well. In Portland, Maine, where I lived for years, drinking alcohol, a legal drug, is the least stigmatized. Smoking cannabis, which is also legal in Maine, has a mixed reputation but is less stigmatized among youth than their parents or grandparents. Injection drug use of any kind is probably the most stigmatized. I once spoke with a woman in recovery from alcohol use disorder who described herself as "just an alcoholic and not an addict."

Across the country, attitudes toward addiction took an unexpected turn in the early 2000s, when young adult white people started dying from overdoses of prescription painkillers (opioids) at alarming rates. By the early 2010s, media descriptions of deaths among rural, poor, "pill seeking" white people gave way to descriptions of young white men looking for prescriptions in their parents' medicine cabinets. These images replaced our stereotypical image of an opioid addict as a Black urban junkie with a needle in his arm. For white middle-class families, opioid addiction and overdose deaths were no longer something that happened somewhere else; for many, they happened at the next-door neighbor's house or even in their own children's bedrooms. Unfortunately, most parents were ashamed and hushed up these deaths. Even after governments and health care providers put measures in place to restrict the number of opioid prescriptions, overdoses continued and increased, primarily among white people. In 2010, the cause of most overdoses was heroin (at the time, it was cheaper than prescription painkillers), and by 2014, fentanyl and other synthetic opioids were the leading cause.[2]

The problem with this narrative of an opioid crisis with white people dying in large numbers is that it's only partly true. The numbers are unquestionably high—too high—but overdose death rates among Black people and Hispanic people have risen dramatically in recent years, too. The age-adjusted rate of overdose deaths for Black people increased 90 times between 1999 and 2017, compared with 39 times for white people and 37 times for Hispanic people. Further, the rise in overdose deaths nationwide during the COVID-19 pandemic received media attention, but not the fact that rates increased significantly among Black people in some regions but decreased among white people.[3] Overall, the media has paid scant attention to rising overdose death rates among people of color.[4]

Data show that nearly half of high school seniors have used cannabis at some point in their lives, and two out of five have been drunk at least once.[5] However, it was opioid use and addiction that propelled stunned parents into calls for action against this "scourge" in their communities. The slogan "addiction doesn't discriminate" became popular as a way to destigmatize addiction. White family members "came out" and talked to policy makers, schools, and the press about their children as bright, happy, and full of life before using drugs. They spoke about their experiences as good, normal parents. They advocated for treatment instead of arrest and incarceration. The statements "Addiction can happen to anyone" and "We can't arrest our way out of this problem" became rallying cries for parents and law enforcement officers who were tired of locking up white kids in their communities. The unspoken message was that "addiction and overdose can even happen in well-to-do white families."

Saying that addiction can happen to anyone may be technically accurate. It conceals, however, the vast and disproportionate burden of addiction in poor communities and among people of color. Intergenerational trauma and social, economic, and political marginalization create risk factors for addiction, and drug policy that isn't uniformly enforced means some people get treatment, and some get incarceration, for the same condition.[6] The reality is that specific populations—people of low socioeconomic status and people of color—are more likely to experience addiction than others.

Social Stigma, Shame, and Discrimination

In 2016, the National Academies of Sciences, Engineering, and Medicine conducted a comprehensive study to understand why stigma around mental health and substance use disorders exists.[7] The study broke stigma into three types: social stigma, self-stigma (shame), and institutional stigma (discrimination).

Social Stigma

This is the negative societal judgment about people with addictions, and it doesn't suddenly evaporate when a person enters recovery. We label, stereotype, exclude, and reject people who have or had a problem with substances. Some of our typical stereotypes of people with addictions (or in recovery) are being dangerous, unpredictable, dishonest, unable to make decisions, and having a bad character. When other conditions are added on—like homelessness or having HIV/AIDS or living in poverty— the stigma increases. Stigma can extend to families of people with addiction, too.[8]

Self-Stigma

Shame happens when people with addiction or in recovery take on the negative judgments of the community as their own. The consequences of shame can be dire. For example, shame about the past is one reason some people start drinking again. Hiding opioid use because of shame creates a considerable risk for overdosing because using alone is a high-risk activity. In addition, people ashamed about their current or past addictions or who felt contempt from health care providers are less likely to seek help or medical care, thereby compromising their long-term health and wellness.

Institutional Stigma

As individuals, people in all walks of life shun people with substance use disorders, and their actions may, in turn, entrench stigma in a variety of institutional and public policies and practices. For example, some employers have policies that punish an individual's drug use by dismissal or turning that person over to law enforcement instead of opening a conversation and offering help and a referral to a health care or treatment provider for an assessment. In the health care system, research shows that patients with substance use disorders receive lower-quality care.[9] In the criminal justice system, discrimination results in the overrepresentation of people with substance use and mental health disorders in America's prisons. Discrimination also results in policy makers being unwilling to commit sufficient resources to support people with addiction and people in recovery.

Stigma and Medications for Addiction

People who take medications for opioid use disorder face discrimination in the recovery community and beyond. Judgmental statements such as,

"They're just trading one drug for another," or "They're not really in recovery," or "It's OK if they're on it for a while, but they should stop as soon as possible" create shame. Sometimes this shame leads people to stop their medications before it's medically safe, and they are at high risk for starting to use again and overdosing. It also leads to secrecy—people hide the fact that they're taking medications from others in the recovery community—when learning how to deal with life honestly is an essential part of living in recovery.

Stigma and Women

Pregnant women who use drugs are the most stigmatized drug and alcohol users, followed closely by women with young children. The shame these women feel about being "bad mothers" can be overwhelming, and they face unique challenges in seeking and maintaining recovery. In addition to learning how to live a life in recovery, women with children need to learn how to parent in recovery. This is sometimes a completely new experience for them. They may have had poor parental role models and not know where to start. They may be in an abusive relationship with their children's father that complicates parenting. They may have underlying physical and mental health issues they need to address before being healthy mothers. Most of all, they fear that they may not be able to comply with treatment recommendations while keeping their family intact or that disclosing their substance use might result in the removal of their children. There is an ongoing fear that they will abruptly lose custody if they relapse during treatment.

Maintaining custody of children (or getting it back) is a powerful motivating factor for women to seek treatment and recovery. Many women benefit from intensive services that include housing, trauma-informed mental health and substance use treatment, job-skill training, school enrollment, childcare, and services for their children, such as play therapy. Supportive relationships with other women and in their own families play an essential role as well.[10]

The Language of Stigma

When asked about the barriers to recovery in his hometown in Massachusetts, Andrew answers, "Stigma, stigma, stigma.

"The language we use as people in recovery, such as the terms 'addict' and 'alco-holic' in our own circles, provokes immediate judgment. Sometimes the health care workers helping us can be judgmental and think we are hopeless. There are libraries full of studies on addiction and few on sustainable long-term recovery. We are ghosts to the rest of the world—there is very little known about long-term, sustainable recovery.

"Stigma reduces a person to nothing more than their difficulties and robs people of possible life opportunities. It leads systems to withhold appropriate treatment and services, and it exposes people to preventable trauma.

"If more people came out and advocated for recovery, stood up for things they believed in, and came out of the dark, a lot of people would see recovery in a different light. Speaking up will get everyday citizens to view the homeless 'junkie' as someone with the potential to get better. More recovery visibility will give communities hope."

Attitudes and beliefs are embedded in the words we use for people with addictions. When we use words like "addict," "lowlife," "junkie," "stoner," "druggie," "dopehead," "drug fiend," "smackhead," and "crackhead," we reinforce the stereotype of untrustworthy, weak, immoral people with criminal intentions. We send a strong message about what we think about people who use drugs and, by extension, people in recovery.[11] These words express our disdain toward people with addictions and contribute to their shame. As one sixty-year-old man in recovery said, "People judge us, and we judge each other by the language we use."

Research shows that when people with addiction feel shame and stigma in the community and at their health care provider's office, they're less likely to seek treatment. When they think staff members stigmatize them in treatment, they're less likely to complete it.[12] Researchers have found that words like "addict," "alcoholic," and "substance abuser" are stigmatizing and have recommended against using them. The current thinking is that person-first language—saying "a person with a substance use disorder" or "a person with a problem with alcohol"—delivers a less harmful message, and many people in the recovery community have adopted this language.[13]

In closed-door meetings, people in 12-step programs introduce themselves as "addicts" or "alcoholics," and sometimes they refer to themselves that way in public. This acknowledgment is an essential tenet of AA: admitting you have a problem and are powerless over it. Some others in recovery and not necessarily part of the 12-step community find it a helpful and critical reminder of where they came from as an "addict" or "alcoholic" and use these terms all the time. Still others in and outside the recovery community choose "addict" or "alcoholic" as a way to reject the "politically correct" use of person-first language.

Research continues about language that hurts and language that helps, and it's hard for people in all fields to keep up with the "right way" to refer to people with addiction and people in recovery. In some communities, the words "addict" and "alcoholic" don't carry the harsh meanings they do in others, so it's important to ask.[14]

FOOD FOR THOUGHT:
STIGMA AND DRUG POLICY

Choosing different language is an important way to reduce stigma. Revising policies toward people who use drugs is another. People who use illegal drugs are criminals, by definition. Law enforcement officers arrest them when they show symptoms of substance use disorder—drug use. The criminalization of drug use has contributed to stigmatizing people who use drugs as criminals, thieves, and ne'er-do-wells, and talking about stigma without mentioning the war on drugs obscures this inconvenient reality. Revamping our drug laws could change that.[15] As a thirty-year-old woman in recovery said, "I was arrested because I was sick. When does that happen with any other disease?"

What Can Allies Do?

Chances are pretty good that, in one way or another, we've all used the stigmatized language associated with addiction, and by extension, with recovery. We may intentionally or unwittingly use language like "addicts," "junkies," or "losers" in settings where they have harsh meanings. We may think that people who start using again "just don't want recovery bad enough" and whisper behind their backs. When we recognize the burden that social stigma imposes on people in active addiction and recovery and change our words and actions, we start to be part of the solution to reducing stigma.

For Everyone

- Examine your attitudes and beliefs about people who use drugs and people who have problems with alcohol. Most of us tend to understand addiction from our own experience, based on what we've seen, how we've been affected, and our own moral compass. Maybe we believe that people who use drugs are selfish because our father had a problem with alcohol and couldn't care for us the way we wanted, or we think that people who use drugs are lazy because our sister spent her days in her room smoking weed and her nights partying with friends and ended up dropping out of school. If we don't have any personal experience, we might be influenced by the media, which bombards us with negative images and language. One way or another, we probably have some negative and outdated attitudes about addiction and recovery that could use an overhaul.

- Reflect on these questions: What experiences in my family, home life, or work life have shaped my attitudes toward people with drug or alcohol problems and people in recovery? Do I think substance use disorder is a disease? A choice? A moral failing? Where can I learn more?

- Open a conversation with your friends, neighbors, and family members about their attitudes toward addiction and recovery.

- Consider using person-first language—that is, "a person with addiction" or "a person with substance use disorder"—and be ready to accept responsibility when you make a mistake or say something that ends up being stigmatizing. Recognize that research constantly updates our knowledge and influences our attitudes, so if recommended language usage changes, be open to changing your language instead of grumbling about it. If you don't know the "right" terminology in a particular situation, it's always a good idea to ask the people you're with, "What's the best way for me to talk about this?"

- Learn more about recovery by reading, attending public events that highlight recovery, and talking with people in recovery. People have negative stereotypes about individuals in recovery because they just don't know much about it.

- Show up at recovery events. September is National Recovery Month, and every year, towns and cities across the country host rallies, marches, and educational opportunities for people to learn about recovery. Attending recovery-related events can send a powerful message to the recovery community that you support their work. It can also send a powerful message to the rest of the community that you aren't afraid to be associated with "those people."

- Call out lousy language and bad attitudes toward people in active use and in recovery when you hear it or see it on a one-to-one, person-to-person basis. You can say something like, "When you say that, it can hurt people trying to change their life. Is that what you meant? Tell me more about why you feel that way."

- Change the conversation. Think about how you talk about addiction and people with problems with drugs or alcohol, and make sure you inject hope into conversations.

  - If someone is making fun of drunk people, change the conversation by saying, "I don't see it that way."

  - If you're in recovery yourself, chime in when someone speaks openly about their recovery by saying, "Me, too." If you're a family member or friend, say something along the lines of "That's great! I know a lot of people in recovery who are doing great things, too."

  - If someone is seeking help, like going to a 12-step meeting, say, "That's great. I've heard that is helpful for a lot of people."

For Community Organizations

- Work with the recovery community to conduct public meetings to educate community members about recovery. Events that combine education about substance use disorder with a person in recovery who talks about their experiences may reduce stigma.

Being in recovery and speaking out about that experience comes with risks and rewards. Ironically, people who come forward and speak at public events about their addiction and recovery to reduce stigma run the risk of being labeled and experiencing discrimination as a result. However, the flip side is that they may also feel less shame and feel a sense of inclusion when their stories elicit empathy and when people in their community listen with compassion. Knowing that speaking out publicly can go either way—reduce or increase shame—it's commendable that so many people in recovery show up and tell their stories.

These events can take place in the community, schools, worksites, faith settings, and anywhere people gather to learn. Public meetings and conversations are important; unfortunately, there is no evidence that these changes in individual attitudes endure in the long term (beyond a month or two), so repeated communication with community members is essential.[16]

Not only do events like community meetings create an opportunity for the community to learn and to meet people in recovery, but they also make connections and new relationships between people in recovery and community members they may not have met before. These connections can open the door to opportunities like employment.

- Conduct a "language audit" of websites, social media, and print materials to ensure language aligns with current research recommendations.

- Work with local media members on the use of language. The *AP Stylebook* recommends using person-first language and avoiding words like "alcoholic" and "addict" unless they are in quotations or names of organizations like the National Institute on Drug Abuse or Alcoholics Anonymous. Community members can get involved by letting local reporters know that using words like "addict" and images of discarded syringes and people injecting drugs in articles about recovery not only stigmatizes recovery but misses an opportunity to present a positive image of recovery. Talking with local reporters and newspaper/television editors about the language and images the press uses should be revisited every year.

For Social Workers, Health Care Providers, and Public Health Professionals

- Ask your clients and patients what they would like you to do to make their recovery journey easier, and be ready to act on it.

- Whenever possible, in public, with family members, in clinical settings, and elsewhere, emphasize that recovery is the most likely outcome for people with substance use disorder.

- Research singles out health care professionals, including mental health counselors, as stigmatizing people who use drugs or are in recovery, perhaps because we expect them to have compassion for everyone, when in fact, they have as many misperceptions about recovery as the rest of us.[17, 18, 19] Recent studies have shown that providing education about addiction and recovery and giving health care providers an opportunity to engage with people in recovery (including attending AA meetings) can change their attitudes.[20]

- Host grand rounds or make a professional presentation with people in recovery and educate your peers about addiction and treatment resources and recovery support services in your area.

- Stay current on your profession's terminology about addiction. Recent research by leading researchers indicates there's no single medical term for "opioid-related impairment" that meets clinical and public health goals. To reduce stigmatizing blame, calling opioid addiction a "chronically relapsing brain disease" may work best; to increase optimism and decrease perceived danger and social exclusion, using nonmedical terminology like "opioid problem" may be best.[21]

- Research shows that the general public responds more positively to people with substance use disorder when it's portrayed as a "treatable illness," so use this terminology when speaking in public meetings.[22]

For Policy Makers

- Research shows that one way to increase the public's willingness to invest in the treatment system is to combine sympathetic personal stories of the difficulties people encounter seeking help with information about the policy issue of structural barriers to substance use treatment.[23]

- There is some evidence that well-crafted communication campaigns can effectively change attitudes, as long as the campaign's goals are clear, and the campaign reaches the intended audience. When diving into an anti-stigma campaign, make sure people in recovery are part of the process. It's probably best to engage a communications specialist who knows how to frame issues and communicate effectively with specific target audiences, too.

10

HARM REDUCTION

ON THE ANNIVERSARY of her thirteenth year in recovery from opioid use disorder, Sarah Siegel—now a healthy mother of three, wife, and ordained interfaith minister—wrote on her Facebook page: "It [the number of years] really could be years more if I looked at my recovery according to the SAMHSA [Substance Abuse and Mental Health Services Administration] definition: 'A process of change through which individuals improve their health and wellness, live a self-directed life, and strive to reach their full potential.'

"When I look back over my journey, I can see that I was engaged in a meaningful process of change for years before I was able to stop using drugs. This is often the case for those healing from addiction: it takes time, and it happens incrementally. This evolving process of change that can completely transform one's life is cause for celebration every step of the way.

"It is normal to be ambivalent in the beginning and at many times throughout the journey. It is normal to know you need to change but not yet know how to make the changes. It is normal to be scared.

"We need to see every step that someone makes in the direction of healing as beautiful, important, and meaningful instead of constantly telling people they aren't doing it 'right.'

"We need to consistently reflect people's inherent goodness and inner strength back to them instead of compounding shame. Shame is what keeps us sick, and shame is what kills.

"Today, I'm honoring the work I've done to get to this place. I'm honoring the work my family has done to heal and to love me through my sickness. Most importantly, on my heart today is remembering all those who have lost their lives to the disease of addiction and asking the Universe to keep supporting me so that I may continue to support others. I am both celebrating the journey thus far and intensely aware that we have much work to do collectively if we want to help others find their way through the darkness of active addiction."

Living and working in the recovery community means confronting death every single day. We've all gotten that call, read that obituary, or had that gut-punched feeling of hearing through the grapevine that someone has died. We've all mourned people who faded away in opioid overdoses and drug-related infections like endocarditis, suffered during the final stages of an alcohol use disorder, or died from strokes after years of stimulant use. Some days it feels like an endless flow of desperate pain and sadness.

Traditionally, harm reduction referred to public health interventions to reduce the adverse risks of intravenous heroin use, such as contracting hepatitis C or HIV. The term has a broader meaning as well. It's what we do to help people who are using drugs and alcohol stay safe while they are using, including preventing overdoses and other actions that people who use drugs take to keep each other alive. Some parents who have lost their children to an overdose and peers who have seen too many friends die have become vocal about harm reduction. What used to be too uncomfortable to talk about has become a vital advocacy issue.

GOT NALOXONE?

Naloxone is a prescription drug that can reverse opioid overdoses if administered soon enough after any type of opioid—prescription pills, heroin, methadone, fentanyl—is ingested. It comes in injection and nasal form. It's harmless for people who don't have any opioids in their system. For people who do have opioids "on board," it blocks brain receptors for those opioids, and when excess opioids have caused breathing to slow or stop, it can restore normal respiration. (If an overdose is caused by a combination of drugs, including an opioid, the naloxone will only temporarily stop the effects of the opioid.) Sometimes, a person who receives naloxone will experience opioid withdrawal symptoms when the naloxone kicks in and the opioid receptors are blocked. The effects of naloxone wear off after 30 to 120 minutes, so if it's safe for you to do so, it's important to call for emergency services after administering it outside a hospital setting.

Some states have passed "Good Samaritan" legislation that protects people who call for emergency services from arrest for possession of drugs or paraphernalia at the site of an overdose. These laws are intended to encourage people who may have drugs in their possession to call for help. The laws vary considerably by state, and enforcement isn't consistent. It's best to learn about the laws and how they are applied in your state.

People who might be present at an overdose, such as other opioid users, staff of recovery residences, and friends and family members of people actively using opioids, should carry naloxone. It can be easy to get, or not, depending on who you are and where you live. State laws govern the distribution of naloxone.[1] Some health care providers will prescribe naloxone as a companion to opioid medication to relieve pain, in case the patient takes too many pain pills and overdoses.

With the increase in opioid overdose deaths and the limited capacity of syringe services programs (SSPs), many State governments, municipalities, and private organizations have stepped in to distribute naloxone to as many people as possible. Pharmacies, health care providers, police departments, recovery community centers, treatment agencies, and recovery residences are just a few places where citizens can get naloxone. Some organizations limit distribution to people at risk for overdose and people who may reverse an overdose, and others take a broader approach and hand it out to anyone who wants it.

What Is Harm Reduction?

Approaches to harm reduction are evolving. Traditional harm reduction programs, syringe services programs (SSPs), include a syringe exchange, where people who inject drugs can turn in used syringes and get new ones and other injecting supplies. These programs also offer free naloxone, the drug that can reverse opioid overdoses. (We don't yet have medicines to reverse overdoses from other drugs, including alcohol.) Some harm reduction programs distribute clean straws for people who snort their drugs, and fentanyl test strips, so people know whether the drug they plan to take contains fentanyl, an opioid responsible for increasing numbers of overdose deaths. Most programs also test for HIV and other sexually transmitted diseases and provide referrals to treatment, social services, and hepatitis treatment clinics. Some programs offer medical care or operate in conjunction with a primary care provider to address problems like skin infections from injecting with unclean needles. Often, they are a safe haven for people in active use, a place free of judgment and full of support, a place where, in the words of one harm reductionist, "we meet people where they're at and don't leave them there."

Harm reduction programs are for people who want to be safer while in active use, make informed decisions with support from staff and peers, or explore ways of increasing safety while not necessarily eliminating drug use. Most people think of injection drug users as people experiencing homelessness or engaging in chronic or compulsive drug use, and indeed some people without permanent housing utilize harm reduction services. But people with secure jobs and families use harm reduction services, too. It comes as a surprise to people outside the harm reduction community that people living stable lives inject drugs and want clean injection supplies.

According to the Drug Policy Alliance, fourteen states have no SSPs, and twelve states have them in one or two cities in the entire state.[2] An outbreak of HIV and hepatitis C in Indiana because of sharing used needles illustrates what can happen when these services aren't available. In early 2015, 135 people actively using drugs in Scott County, Indiana, tested positive for HIV; most were also diagnosed with hepatitis C. Following contact tracing, an additional 109 tested positive for HIV. To put this in perspective, before the outbreak, the county had seen fewer than five HIV cases annually. Residents and public health professionals were ill-prepared to respond. SSPs had long been banned in Indiana, and it took the declaration of a public health emergency and new legislation in March 2015 to allow SSPs to operate.[3] The SSP in Scott County produced results: there were just seven new HIV cases in 2019. Lawmakers didn't understand the long-term importance of harm reduction, though. In June 2021, the Scott County commissioners voted to close the program on January 1, 2022.[4]

Harm reduction programs are highly stigmatized. Some people think that giving people injection supplies encourages drug use even though there's no scientific evidence to back up that viewpoint. Nearly thirty years of research have shown SSPs to be safe, effective, and cost-saving. They don't increase illegal drug use or crime. They play an essential role in reducing the transmission of viral hepatitis, HIV, and other infections, and they often serve as a bridge to treatment for people who use their services.[5] Even with a wealth of research supporting the effectiveness of SSPs, the US government hasn't consistently supported them. It took the shock of the Scott County public health crisis for federal lawmakers to pass legislation authorizing federal funding for SSPs, with the exception of purchasing needles.[6]

Overdose Prevention Sites

Overdose prevention sites, also called safe use facilities, supervised injection sites, or safe injection sites, are a new way to promote safer drug use. These settings allow people to take their drugs and use them with health care providers, harm reductionists, and peers nearby. The health care provider can administer naloxone to reverse an overdose, if necessary, or address other medical situations that may arise. Referrals to treatment and other services are available, too. Overdose prevention sites are currently illegal in the United States, although informal, underground sites exist. A literature review of research, mostly from sites in Australia and Canada, shows that they promote safer injection conditions, enhance access to primary care, and reduce overdoses. They don't result in increased drug trafficking or crime in the surrounding area, and they're associated with less public injecting and fewer improperly disposed-of syringes.[7] Harm reductions in the United States are testing the legality of overdose prevention sites, including the opening of two overdose prevention centers in New York City.[8]

Harm Reduction and Social Justice

I met Jesse in the early months of his recovery when he left Massachusetts and came to Portland, Maine, for a fresh start. We attended public meetings together around Maine, where he told his story. Jesse's recovery was initially grounded in abstinence and AA, and his story was a traditional narrative of struggles with addiction, mental health challenges, and hopes in recovery. Jesse sought training as a peer navigator in a local health center that served marginalized people all over Portland. In that role, Jesse reached out to people in the shadows as well as helped all others he met in all walks of life. (Jesse also helped me personally to find treatment for a close friend.) He quit his job to pursue a master's degree in public policy at the University of Southern Maine. While there he worked at the Recovery Oriented Campus Center.

Jesse created and ran four low-barrier recovery residences for people without much money in two towns that were notorious for their drug problems. Municipal officials were hostile to the presence of recovery housing, and he successfully educated them about the requirements of the Fair Housing Act to keep the houses open. Jesse opened the first women's house that allowed medications for addiction in a southern Maine county. He sought and received Maine Association of Recovery Residences (MARR) certification for all of his houses, even though that was not a requirement for operating them. With these low-barrier houses that accepted medications for addiction, Jesse changed the paradigm for recovery housing in Maine, and now more houses, including houses for LGBTQIA+ and returning citizens (ex-prisoners), are being opened using his model. All of the houses he started are now thriving.

As Jesse grew in the spirit of recovery, his story changed. He rejected abstinence as the only path to recovery. He moved away from that model and advocated for policy change that would have a beneficial effect on more people. He despaired of mainstream actions to increase access to naloxone as the primary intervention to prevent overdose deaths, saying, "All the naloxone in the world won't stop overdoses." Jesse became known across the nation for founding the Church of Safe Injection that was rooted in "radical compassion" for people who use drugs, sex workers, and people experiencing homelessness or poverty, and he believed the First Amendment should protect his actions. Through the church, he distributed naloxone, clean injection supplies, and fentanyl test strips and food and clothing out of his car until law enforcement put a stop to it. (The Church of Safe Injection wasn't a state-approved syringe services program at the time but has since received that designation.[9]) Jesse was a founding member of the Portland Overdose Prevention Society and became an outspoken advocate for safe injection sites, drug user unions, and human rights for people who use drugs.

"People who use drugs don't deserve to die," was Jesse's mantra. He followed his passion even when it wasn't easy. He took on law enforcement, politicians, bureaucrats,

and church leaders, and he inspired hundreds of harm reductionists who continue to carry his message. Sadly, like many committed harm reduction advocates before him, facing daily struggles, he died from a drug overdose in 2020. He was twenty-eight. Jesse's work took root and continues to thrive through the hundreds of people he inspired.

Jesse isn't the only person who was outspoken about the human rights of people who use drugs. In the past few years, harm reductionists from organizations such as the National Harm Reduction Coalition, the Chicago Recovery Alliance, and local and regional drug user unions have formed a social justice movement founded on this principle. They support people who use drugs being able to make their own informed decisions about how they want to live while also acknowledging the harms that using drugs can cause, and they promote people who use drugs helping each other and the formation of drug user unions.

The new harm reduction movement has issued a call for the rights of people who use drugs and demands a seat for them at the table when drug issues are discussed. The movement has also called for an end to the national war on drugs, which President Nixon officially launched in 1971 and which radically changed drug sentencing laws and increased the size of federal law enforcement agencies. Now most drug violation arrests are for possession (not trafficking), so people who are using drugs and people with addictions often end up in jail or prison. Appropriate treatment and support are rarely available during incarceration. People with felony convictions can be denied housing, education, and employment, so our punitive drug policy creates stigma and discrimination that last a lifetime. Drug policy in the United States contributes to a cycle of separated families, childhood trauma (due to having an incarcerated parent), and entrenched poverty that are conditions for initiating drug use. The people most affected are people of color and people with mental health issues. The reverberating effect on families and communities is immense.[10]

Ending the war on drugs could mean legalizing or decriminalizing all substances. Some states are moving in this direction with the legalization of cannabis and psilocybin (the psychedelic compound in some mushrooms). It could mean changing drug sentencing laws, so that possession of small amounts results in an offer for help and treatment instead of a prison sentence. It could also mean ending racialized drug policies, including the unequal enforcement of existing drug laws that have landed far more people of color in jail and prison than white people and resulted in enormous harm in communities of color.[11]

Moderate Use and Plant-Based Recovery

Sarah F. was in and out of treatment and recovery in her late teens and early twenties, including attending 12-step meetings. When she moved to Maine from Michigan and found out she was pregnant, she stopped using all drugs, including heroin. Her husband was still using, so he was "super sick," and she was "super sober" for the first time in years. "As a new mom with a husband who wasn't doing well, I was driven to learn more about harm reduction, to apply it to my own family," she explained. She wanted to help her husband, and she didn't believe in AA's abstinence-only approach anymore. She met some people who smoked cannabis, and after her pregnancy she decided she'd do it and be open about it. Around the same time, she connected with people who supported her recovery, even though it wasn't abstinence-based. "That's what pushed me into harm reduction," she said.

Sarah has a history of PTSD (post-traumatic stress disorder), depression, and anxiety, and she didn't want to go the route of prescribed medications. "That works for some people, but I had some experiences with antidepressants before, and I just didn't want to do that." She and her husband started growing cannabis. "It was a really beautiful process, with unexpected moments of healing," she explained. "Some women want a man to bring them flowers. My husband grows me plants, grows me my medicine! It's really cool to see him involved in that process and to see our kids involved, too, in watering and taking care of the plants."

Sarah and her husband use psilocybin, too. They did research and talked with people who had used it and decided they wanted to give it a try. They both found that cannabis and psilocybin helped with depression and anxiety and generally helped them work together as parents. "Speaking as a parent," Sarah says, "there's so much research on the negative effect that parents' drug use has on kids. But what about the opposite? Cannabis allows me to relax. Instead of navigating panic attacks, I'm able to connect more authentically with my children. After microdosing psilocybin, I'm much happier, much more present in the moment as a parent."

She believes in both pharmaceuticals and naturally occurring substances. "I think there needs to be a world where there is access to both. Plants and psychedelic medications are so stigmatized; so much misinformation is spread about them," Sarah says. "There's so much potential. And besides, who am I to judge about how people want to heal?"

Some people in recovery turn to moderate use, either of the drug they were addicted to or another substance. For some people with histories of severe addiction, this may be a dangerous gamble. On the other hand, people with a mild or moderate substance use disorder may find that they can use drugs in moderation without significant negative consequences. Research indicates that people with a less severe drinking problem and a high degree of confidence in reducing the times of heavy drinking may be able to drink in moderation.[12] People who attempt to drink in moderation and aren't successful are at high risk for a return to active addiction.[13]

Some people recovering from addiction to one drug find it safe to use another drug or drugs, sometimes called being "California sober." For example, a person with an opioid addiction in the past may smoke cannabis without any harmful results. While anecdotally this may be the case, no scientific studies confirm it, and research is underway. Similarly, anecdotal information from people in recovery suggests that using psychedelics is helpful for some people in stable recovery.

TREATMENT, HARM REDUCTION, RECOVERY, OR BAD POLICY?

The recovery community isn't united in its views on medications for addiction. Methadone treatment for opioid addiction has traditionally been considered a harm reduction strategy since the Food and Drug Administration (FDA) approved its use in 1972. When the FDA added buprenorphine formulations (Suboxone) in 2002, many people viewed it as harm reduction as well. Those who take methadone or Suboxone for years and regain employment and family connections see them as treatment for a chronic disease and part of a healthy recovery.

Health care providers have set up innovative programs in emergency rooms to prescribe Suboxone to patients who have overdosed, reducing the chances of another overdose, and so emergency rooms are a new setting for incorporating harm reduction strategies. Not everyone thinks this is a good idea, however, because hospitals and emergency rooms usually can't provide other support services and basic needs. Some advocates believe that sending a person who has recently overdosed out the door with a packet of Suboxone and a referral to treatment is irresponsible and insufficient, especially for people with few resources or who are without housing. They point to the disaster of Boston's "Methadone Mile," where scores of people without housing or other services congregate in an open-air drug market adjacent to addiction services (methadone and Suboxone) to buy and sell all kinds of drugs. People in Philadelphia's Kensington district and the Blade in Seattle have suffered this same fate, where state and federal policies make resources available for medications but aren't sufficient for housing, mental health services, and recovery support services.

Harm Reduction and Recovery

People in the recovery community don't universally support harm reduction. Some see traditional harm reduction (syringe exchanges and overdose prevention) as a "free pass" to use drugs. For many who consider abstinence essential to recovery, a person receiving harm reduction services isn't "really in recovery." For people who believe that "you have to hit rock bottom" before real recovery starts, harm reduction might delay that step to getting better. There's also a fear in the recovery community about sending the wrong message about using drugs or alcohol, even in moderation. Opponents of using in moderation as a harm reduction strategy want to protect people who can't use any amount of alcohol or drugs safely. Some people are uneasy about calling for an end to the war on drugs for this reason, too.

But in a way that is seldom discussed, recovery is harm reduction. Sometimes, seeing hope in the lives of people in recovery acts as a light in the dark for people who are in active addiction, and as a result some use less or take steps toward better health. Other times, keeping connected with a supportive community prevents people in recovery from using again. Carolyn Delaney, publisher of the Portland, Maine–based *Journey Magazine* that amplifies hope for recovery, says, "It breaks my heart that addiction is more visible than recovery." Visible recovery *is* harm reduction when people learn about the possibility of recovery and try it out for themselves. Visible recovery can save lives.

Attitudes in the recovery community have shifted considerably in recent years. Young people who accessed harm reduction services as part of their path to recovery are now a vocal part of the recovery community. They've seen too many of their friends die from overdoses and have opened a dialogue with their peers in recovery. They see a clear need to advocate to protect people who aren't using in moderation. Parents who lost their children to opioid overdoses have also become a loud voice for harm reduction services in their communities. The result is a shift from opposition to tolerance and, in some cases, acceptance of harm reduction as an essential service. Some have gone a step further and include "any positive change" in their definition of recovery. Like Sarah Siegel, who posted about her recovery on Facebook, they see every effort made in the direction of healing as "beautiful, important, and meaningful." This approach creates the radical notion that supporting harm reduction is love. For some harm reductionists, it merges two opposite worlds—harm reduction and recovery—into one: harm reduction and recovery are both processes moving toward greater health and connection and are the same.

What Can Allies Do?

As hard as it is for some people to accept, drug use is a fact of life in our country, and opioid overdose deaths are a tragic part of everyday life. As much as we might want abstinence for the people we love, we need to accept that keeping them alive is more important than imposing our ideas on them. To do our part in preventing disease and death due to substance use, we can support individuals who practice harm reduction, community harm reduction programs that distribute clean syringes, supplies, and naloxone, and statewide efforts to distribute naloxone and increase access to treatment. Recreational and medical cannabis are legal in many states, making it easier to use them than in the past. Supporting moderate use of cannabis or alcohol or any drug may be a difficult pill to swallow for many, but if it keeps people alive, it's worth it.

For Everyone

- Carry naloxone! Find out where to get naloxone in your community and learn how to use it. Harm reduction organizations, pharmacies, health care providers, police departments, recovery community centers, treatment agencies, and recovery residences are just a few places where citizens can get naloxone and receive training in when and how to administer it.

- Explore your own attitudes about harm reduction. If it has made you uncomfortable in the past, you may find that you can learn about the continuum of drug use and why people use drugs and appreciate the changes they make toward wellness, even if they aren't the changes you'd like to see or that seem logical or reasonable to you.

- Find out what harm reduction services are in your area. Then you'll be ready to support someone who wants to reduce harm while they're using drugs.

- Seek out advocacy opportunities in your community and state to reduce the stigma of harm reduction and prevent overdose deaths.

For Community Organizations

- Hold naloxone trainings in your community. You can do this by reaching out to a recovery center or harm reduction program nearby and asking them to come and teach people about how to use naloxone, if your state permits it.

- Look for opportunities to increase access to naloxone. Some advocates look to organizations like colleges and universities and large employers to add a "NaloxBox" next to the automated external defibrillator (AED), so lifesaving naloxone is available just like a lifesaving defibrillator.

For Health Care Providers

- Explore the possibility of prescribing naloxone to family members and friends, as well as individuals who are at risk for overdose, and build in reminders in the electronic medical record.

- Make sure you know about risks associated with injection drug use like abscesses and endocarditis, and also wound care and harm reduction services in your area and refer your patients. Tell family members about them, too.

- Consider volunteering at syringe services programs or naloxone distribution organizations.

- Talk with your patients about their harm reduction practices and ask what they would like you to do to support them.

RECOVERY, TRAUMA, AND MENTAL ILLNESS

RECOVERY ALLIES IS about the successes people have had in finding and sustaining recovery on their terms; it's not about what doesn't work. However, sometimes the recovery journey gets rocky, and substance use treatment and recovery support services don't help. Neither was designed to address mental health conditions or trauma, which are common in people with addiction. In my interviews with people in recovery, trauma related to sexual abuse in childhood, incarceration as a child or an adult, and the aftereffects of taking psychotropic medications to address mental health conditions in childhood frequently came up. (I didn't interview any veterans, so I don't include combat experience, which creates another unique form of trauma exposure.)

Understanding trauma is an entire field of study, and I bring it up here in the context of the difficulties past trauma can create for people in recovery. Several people I interviewed with histories of trauma talked openly about their experiences in Alcoholics Anonymous as being more harmful than helpful. Because AA is foundational to recovery in the United States, and to honor their journeys, I feel it is important to include them in the book. We've seen that AA can help people get sober, stay sober, drink less, and suffer fewer consequences of drinking, so we know it is effective for some people, including people who have experienced trauma; it's just not helpful for everyone.

Cynthia had been in and out of recovery for twenty-one years. She had attended 12-step meetings for her problems with alcohol and painkillers, but when her partner committed suicide, the extreme trauma created a significant and unexpected change in direction in her recovery journey. She continued going to AA, but says she felt like a fish out of water now. When she talked about her partner's death, it felt like almost everyone avoided her. Only one woman reached out with compassion. Cynthia realized she needed a type of support she didn't find in the halls of Alcoholics Anonymous.

For Cynthia and many like her, "working the fourth step"—making a "searching and fearless moral inventory" of herself—caused her to revisit the suicide again and again and was retraumatizing. "There's no support for people in AA who have gone through extreme trauma," Cynthia says. "What's your part in your experience? You're supposed to answer that question. People in AA told me, 'You chose someone with a brain injury. You knew something like this could happen.' They all said the reason for anything that happened was because I was an alcoholic, but that just wasn't true."

Cynthia quit going to AA meetings and "went alternative," which for her meant learning deep breathing, doing water aerobics, having acupuncture treatments, and practicing yoga. She went to a psychiatrist who practiced the Emotional Freedom Technique (EFT), a type of acupressure, also called tapping, that restores the equilibrium to energies in the body. The psychiatrist helped her acknowledge her trauma, which also really helped her, and told her, "There's no medication out there for this kind of extreme trauma."

"In AA, they say that if you stop going to meetings, you will drink again. But I didn't," Cynthia says. "Organically, after my partner's death, all these people started coming into my life who have experienced trauma, like people who were suicide survivors. My world got bigger and deeper in a way I never thought was possible. I was so enmeshed in AA that I felt like that was the only way I could live. If I left it, I would drink or hang around people who would drink, and then I'd be a lone wolf, and I wouldn't have anything. I stuck with AA out of desperation. Now I realize that I'm OK without AA. I'm not going to drink. I have all these modalities that help me.

"I thought that there was nothing else for me except AA. But there is so much out there that is helpful. It doesn't need to be treatment or alcohol related. It can be counseling, yoga, or just hanging out with people I trust and feel safe with."

Cynthia acknowledges that each AA meeting is different and that she was in a rural area with few options. The people in the meeting she went to were of the "pull yourself up by the bootstraps" variety. But she feels that AA's approach to recovery doesn't work for people coping with extreme trauma. "The people who have the loudest voices have been helped by AA, and the people who have the softest voices have been harmed by it," she says. "Something needs to change. AA doesn't help with trauma, and doctors who prescribe brain-altering drugs don't help either. People with trauma and addiction need connection. How do we get it for them?"

Trauma

Trauma happens when a person experiences or witnesses something that is psychologically overwhelming. As with recovery, researchers continue to refine our understanding and definition of trauma. For now, the Substance Abuse and Mental Health Services Administration defines individual trauma as "an event, series of events, or set of circumstances that is experienced by an individual as physically or emotionally harmful or life threatening and that has lasting adverse effects on the individual's functioning and mental, physical, social, emotional, or spiritual wellbeing."[1] Less formally, trauma is an emotional wound resulting from a single shocking occurrence like living through a hurricane; repeated incidents like bullying, sexual abuse, or combat; or ongoing circumstances like childhood neglect and abandonment. Intergenerational trauma is a form of collective trauma, when an event in the past—like genocide or forced dislocation—created trauma in large numbers of individuals who then transmit it to their children through their own psychological responses of dread, worry, and despair.

Everyone responds differently to trauma, and people may need specialized treatment in addition to care and compassion.[2] Researchers have drawn a clear connection between trauma and addiction: People who have experienced trauma are more likely to develop substance use disorders. Researchers recognize that addressing trauma through a "trauma-informed" approach to treatment and health care is crucial in helping people heal.[3]

Faye, who suffered sexual abuse as a child, says she gained a new understanding of herself when a psychiatrist explained that complex childhood trauma can cause changes in the brain's structure and functioning that in turn affect future development. "I learned that this may lead to having a hard time coping with everyday life and difficulties with concentration and memory. It can also lead to challenges in having stable relationships. Many people with complex trauma turn to drugs or alcohol to cope.

"Trauma is a 'thing' now, where everyone has some sort of trauma in their lives," Faye says. *"We've cheapened the term. For people with real trauma, the consequences are enormous. It's a brain injury that affects every aspect of my life. Community members need to be aware that many people with substance use disorder have trauma in their backgrounds. They need to understand that trauma is an actual brain injury. And we're talking real trauma—not like it's used so widely in public, which is a diminishment of people who have real trauma. People in the community don't even know when they are doing this."*

The Pair of ACEs

Research has identified specific experiences in childhood that can result in trauma and chronic stress—adverse childhood experiences (ACEs)—and conditions in communities that create conditions for trauma—adverse community environments (also ACEs, hence the phrase "pair of ACEs" that is used to refer to the two together). Research shows that adverse childhood experiences can impact a child's developing brain and lead to high-risk behaviors like drug and alcohol use and chronic diseases like diabetes and heart disease. People with more adverse childhood experiences in their past and people living in adverse community environments have higher risks for chronic illnesses, including substance use disorder.

Adverse childhood experiences include:[4]

- Emotional abuse

- Physical abuse

- Sexual abuse

- Emotional neglect

- Physical neglect

- Caregiver treated violently

- Household substance abuse

- Household mental illness

- Parental separation or divorce

- Incarcerated household member

New research on adverse community environments tends to focus on urban environments. It points to communities with high levels of violence as a root cause of widespread individual trauma that results in collective trauma. Characteristics of adverse community environments include:[5]

- Intergenerational poverty
- Long-term unemployment
- Relocation of businesses and jobs
- Limited employment
- Disinvestment
- Deteriorated and dangerous public spaces
- Unhealthy food options
- Disconnected and damaged social relations and networks
- Destructive social norms
- Low sense of collective political and social efficacy

Trauma and the 12 Steps

Like many recovery supports, what works for one person doesn't work for another. Many people with trauma in their past find strength and support in Alcoholics Anonymous and other 12-step programs. Others don't and find AA's fourth step, doing the "searching and fearless moral inventory," particularly damaging. The idea behind this step is for members to gain a clear understanding of themselves, their character, and weaknesses that may have contributed to their alcohol problems. Usually, they work with a sponsor, who helps them accept responsibility for "their part" of their past.[6]

For some people, talking about the trauma and accepting "their part" doesn't make sense. In Cynthia's case, she thought it was absurd to believe that her choice of a partner is "her part" in the traumatic event of his suicide. Similarly, it's hard to imagine how adults can accept "their part" of childhood abuse and neglect or any other adverse childhood event. Just talking about trauma can be retraumatizing if it's not done right, and well-intentioned people with no training in trauma-informed care or experience of their own may inflict harm. One woman I spoke with had been sexually abused at the age of three by her father. Her male sponsor asked her to "consider her part" by trying to understand how angry and disturbed her father must have been to abuse his child. The sponsor urged her to show empathy toward her father. This resulted in the woman returning to using heroin for a short time.

Jamie Marich, a trauma treatment specialist, person in long-term recovery, and author of *Trauma and the 12 Steps: An Inclusive Guide to Enhancing Recovery*, provides a different perspective. She acknowledges the harm that 12-step programs have caused, especially when sponsors present the steps as rigid "absolute orders" rather than guides to recovery. She finds healing mechanisms in the 12-step approach, when it's applied with flexibility, like finding networks of support from other people in recovery and hearing others share similar stories of past trauma that convey the message "You're not alone." For therapists, she maintains that evidence-based interventions are important, but it's the therapeutic alliance—the positive relationship between the clinician and the client—that heals. Clinicians can help prepare clients for the fourth step by helping resolve past trauma before taking on that moral inventory. Working alongside the client to build recovery capital is part of the clinician's job, and 12-step meetings can be part of that.[7]

Mental Illness

About 40 percent of people with substance use disorder also have some co-occurring mental health condition, including anxiety, depression, attention-deficit/hyperactivity disorder, borderline personality disorder, bipolar disorders, or schizophrenia. About half of the people who experience a mental illness during their lives will also experience a substance use disorder and vice versa. Research indicates that 43 percent of people in substance use treatment for nonmedical use of prescription painkillers have a diagnosis or symptoms of mental health disorders, particularly depression and anxiety, and 30–60 percent of people seeking treatment for alcohol use disorder have post-traumatic stress disorder (PTSD) symptoms.[8, 9]

People with these co-occurring issues often find their needs aren't met by addressing their substance use alone. Stopping the use of substances can unleash difficult emotions that they're not equipped to manage. Some, like Faye, find the insights of a good psychiatrist helpful. Others, like Cynthia, seek alternative supports. Many people say that having friendships full of trust and support is the best "medicine."

Medications for Mental Health Conditions

Medications for mental health conditions can be lifesaving, and many people benefit from them. Others suffer ill effects from them, sometimes for a lifetime. For people like Cynthia, the ill effects of antipsychotic drugs, ADHD drugs, antianxiety drugs, and medications for addiction created a distrust of pharmaceutical companies and their profit motives. Many of these "psychiatric survivors" don't want to recover to the younger person they were. They want to resist the forces that created the addictive behaviors in the first place.

What Can Allies Do?

For Everyone

- When someone tells you they have trauma, believe them. Everyone's experience is different, and not everyone who has experienced a traumatic event ends up with trauma or PTSD. But rarely in serious conversation will someone say they've been traumatized when it's not true.

- Saying something was "so traumatic" when you're referring to a difficult situation that then resolved makes people who have truly experienced trauma feel like their experience has been cheapened or lessened. When you say you've experienced "trauma," make sure it fits the definition of trauma: "Individual trauma is an event, series of events, or set of circumstances that is experienced by an individual as physically or emotionally harmful or life threatening and that has lasting adverse effects on the individual's functioning and mental, physical, social, emotional, or spiritual wellbeing."

- One important element in healing from trauma is developing consistently supportive networks of people. This could be in relationships at work, at school, in the family, or in the community. Even social relationships that consist of small talk can be supportive. According to one trauma expert, "More than anything else, being able to feel safe with other people defines mental health; safe connections are fundamental to meaningful and satisfying lives."[10] You may be able to create some safe connections and support for people with a history of trauma.

- Don't assume you "know what it's like," and don't make comments like, "Well, at least you survived." Use active listening and say supportive things like, "Thank you for sharing your very difficult experience with me."

For Social Workers and Health Care Providers

- Learn about trauma-informed care in your field and find ways to educate your peers about it.
- Look for resources in your town or region like support groups that can help people with mental health and trauma.

SECTION 4
The Pillars of Recovery: Health

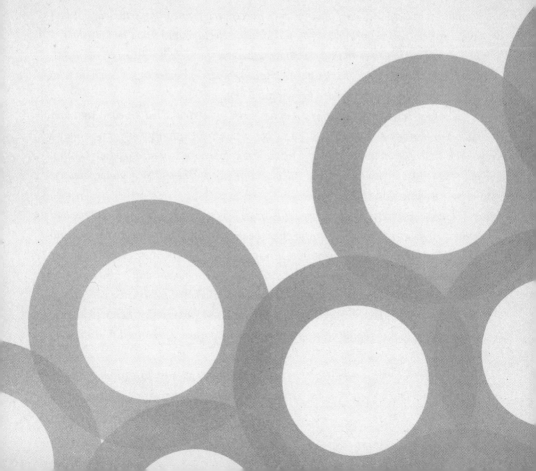

12

HEALTH AND WELLNESS

"WHEN I FIRST entered recovery, I had a LOT of health problems," Carolyn says. Carolyn is in her fifties now and has been in recovery for nearly thirty years. "I had a bad spleen. I had a urinary tract and kidney infection, and I had bad eyesight. I had so many problems, and I didn't know where to start." At her recovery residence, Carolyn's case manager steered her to a primary care provider at a free clinic who helped her identify what needed to be treated first.

The case manager suggested an optometrist, who conducted an eye exam and gave Carolyn glasses for free. "Before I got glasses, everything was fuzzy. I didn't realize that it shouldn't have been fuzzy. I didn't realize I needed glasses. Getting glasses really changed my world. I still go to this guy, twenty-six years later, because he gave us girls at the house free eye care.

"I did some pretty crazy things while I was using, and the people around me had some serious questions about my mental health. You know, in early sobriety and even in active alcoholism, mental health is so subjective. Because of my behavior and my family history of bipolar, I was diagnosed with bipolar and ended up in the psych ward for an inpatient stay after about a year in recovery. Several years later, I got the flu and stopped taking the medications because I was so sick. I didn't have the emotional swings without the medication, and the doctors determined that I wasn't bipolar.

"Is it mental or physical?" Carolyn asks. "In recovery, it's easy to attribute physical ailments to mental conditions. For example, about eight to ten years into recovery, I

had pernicious anemia caused by a vitamin B12 deficiency, a vitamin D deficiency, and iron-deficiency anemia—symptoms from each of them resembled depression. But I had a physical problem in addition to a mental health challenge."

Carolyn's message for other people in recovery is: *"Have a really good health care doctor, and don't just assume that symptoms of depression mean you're depressed!"*

The consequences of an unhealthy and chaotic lifestyle in addiction can reverberate for years, but the good news is that the body heals, and many health problems recede or disappear. After taking care of issues in the first year or two of recovery, people talk about achieving heightened physical energy, improved mental health, and a renewed zest for living. When they reach the five-year milestone of recovery—medically, five years of remission from substance use disorder—their chances of having an active addiction again are about the same as for the general population.[1, 2]

Simply removing drugs or alcohol isn't like waving a magic wand, and all of a sudden, health and wellness appear. Getting well takes time and effort, and the more substances and the longer they were used, the more significant the challenges and the longer it may take to get healthy. The more we know about the difficulties people in recovery are facing, the more we can support them.

Health Consequences of Addiction

Early Recovery

In the first year or two of recovery, people may have some especially tough health challenges. When they stop using drugs, clearheadedness doesn't come all at once. Lurking mental health problems like depression and anxiety can surface. Fatigue, irritability, and brain fog may set in as the brain starts to heal. The quantity of drugs used and duration of use influence how long it takes for a person's brain to clear, and it could be many months or even years. If a person used drugs or alcohol to help them sleep, they might battle insomnia, nightmares, and night sweats when they first stop using. These can be especially frustrating when navigating the new world of recovery, and the one thing that they have relied on most to cope—drugs or alcohol—is gone.

Every health issue is important, but there typically are a few key problems to check out ASAP, and then a plan can be developed for taking care of less-pressing issues. Trying to address all health problems at the same time—stop drinking, quit smoking, exercise, eat a healthy diet, and more—might be a little ambitious.

The first step in tackling health problems is to get a primary care provider (PCP), someone who can look at the "whole person" and figure out what needs to be addressed first. If you're lucky, you'll find a PCP who has addiction or mental health counselors on staff and on site. (This is sometimes called "integrated care.") If you don't have access to a PCP, you can still start by dealing with acute health problems like infections, unfilled cavities, and sexually transmitted diseases as the first priority. Mental health issues that drugs and alcohol have hidden need to be addressed as well, and that might require seeking out a psychiatrist, pastor, counselor, traditional healer, or peer support. Later, maintaining recovery requires ongoing checkups for any chronic problems like diabetes, cancer screenings, and paying close attention to overall physical and emotional wellness.[3]

For people who aren't interested in conventional medicine and prefer other healing practices like ayurvedic medicine or acupuncture, it's important to find a trusted practitioner who can figure out what health issues need to be taken care of and follow progress. Many people prefer a combination of conventional medicine and other ways of healing to meet the health problems they experience.

Physical Health

The short-term and long-term consequences of excessive, chronic drug and/or alcohol use include cancers of the bladder, colon, esophagus, lungs, mouth and throat, pancreas, and stomach. Injecting drugs can lead to HIV, hepatitis, and other infectious diseases. Smoking any drug damages the respiratory system. Most drugs, including alcohol, can wreak havoc on the cardiovascular system.[4,5,6,7,8] People in early recovery often have unfilled cavities and missing teeth.[9]

For many people, physical health in recovery isn't just about the effects on their bodies of using drugs or alcohol for years. People with severe mental illness like schizophrenia and people who have survived childhood trauma face increased risk for diabetes, cardiovascular disease, cancer, and other diseases. People who have survived trauma may experience chronic stress and significant changes in their brains and are at risk for these diseases as well.[10,11]

Tobacco Use

People with addictions are especially affected by tobacco use—they smoke more than most other people, and using tobacco together with alcohol or drugs increases the risk of smoking-related diseases compared with using any one of those substances alone. It might come as a surprise that people treated for alcohol or drug addiction are more likely to die from smoking-related diseases than from causes related to their alcohol or drug use. Medical research is clear that quitting smoking is essential for long-term health, and although people with addictions are just as interested as other people in quitting smoking, cessation services are hard to come by in treatment settings, recovery residences, and recovery community centers.[12, 13, 14, 15, 16, 17]

Mental Health

People with addictions are about twice as likely to have a mood or anxiety disorder.[18] Substance use disorders also occur with schizophrenia, bipolar disorders, ADHD, borderline personality disorder, and antisocial personality disorder.[19] Untreated, these conditions create challenges for a robust recovery. Medications may work for some people, but not everyone. A lifetime of prescribed psychiatric medications—often starting in early childhood—creates difficult lifelong consequences that lead some people to call themselves "psychiatric survivors."

Long-Term Recovery

People in long-term recovery face the same health and wellness challenges as the rest of us, with some important exceptions. The National Recovery Survey (NRS), conducted in 2016, allowed researchers to understand for the first time the ongoing burden of physical disease in people in long-term recovery.[20] The results found that alcohol-related illnesses occurred long after drinking had stopped, and rates of hepatitis C, chronic obstructive pulmonary disease, heart disease, and diabetes were higher for people in recovery than other adults. The same may be true of HIV/AIDS.

Pain Management

Ron is in his late sixties and is in recovery from opioid use disorder. Over the years, he's had numerous hospitalizations and operations, including six spinal fusion surgeries, that required exposure to opioids. For him—and others with a past opioid addiction—one of the core challenges in recovery is managing pain, especially chronic pain, without resorting to opioid painkillers. "I have tried almost every type of pain-management method and strategy," Ron says. "A few were effective, especially meditation with a special focus on chronic pain issues. I studied mindfulness before the word became popularized! I started Botox injections to reduce the frequency of migraines and learned to ask for substitutes for opiates when at the hospital. Now I receive low-dose ketamine instead of opioids for migraines, kidney stones, or whatever presents."

Ron has found a sympathetic primary care provider (PCP) who has been very helpful. He has been upfront with his PCP about his past opioid addiction and opened the door to fruitful conversations about dealing with pain. His PCP referred him to a pain clinic and a psychologist who specializes in chronic pain relief. Sometimes the complex protocol of managing his pain includes pain medication for a short time. "When that happens," Ron says, "I have learned to be open and accountable with my doctor and my partner."

People in recovery from opioid use disorder face particular challenges in managing acute and chronic pain. Some people don't seek help for their pain because they're afraid they'll start misusing opioids or other drugs again if the doctor offers them opioid painkillers. Others are afraid they'll start using drugs again if their pain isn't adequately treated. Still others worry that doctors won't take their pain seriously or will accuse them of drug-seeking behavior. Some on medication for opioid addiction (Suboxone or methadone) are afraid of withdrawal if they don't receive that medication on time.[21] Some who had an addiction to prescription drugs are suspicious of or downright disgusted with the American health care system and aren't inclined to seek help from the same doctors who prescribed them opioids in the first place.

Untreated pain can be a downramp for returning to drug or alcohol use, so managing it is a top priority. Hospitals and health care systems have pain-management specialists. Federal agencies have protocols for treating pain that include strict prescribing guidelines for opioids and other drugs.[22,23] Therapeutic exercise, physical therapy, and cognitive behavioral therapy are nonpharmacological solutions accepted by mainstream health care providers. Many people in recovery seek holistic avenues like acupuncture, yoga, massage, and meditation.

Access to Health Care

People in active addiction have worse health outcomes, are more likely to experience discrimination and stigma in the doctor's office or hospital, and often receive second-rate care compared with people without a severe substance use disorder.[24] When they enter recovery, they continue to experience stigma and sometimes don't seek health care when they need it for that reason.

In the United States, treatment systems for substance use and mental health have operated in separate universes of reimbursement, standards, and access, even though mental illness and addiction occur together as frequently as they occur independently.[25] Physical health care occupies a world of its own as well. When people in and seeking recovery use services from these different systems, they often receive uncoordinated, ineffective care.[26] It's not unusual for an emergency room doctor to be unaware that a patient is on methadone or for a PCP not to know that a patient is participating in counseling or 12-step meetings. Given the unique health care needs of people in recovery, this doesn't result in optimal health care.

While some states and cities have implemented recovery-oriented systems of care and recovery management, treatment and health care systems have historically had little ongoing monitoring, support, or meaningful linkages to peer support and the broader community after treatment or health care is complete. This isn't a recipe for supporting long-term recovery.[27]

Insurance Coverage for Treatment

People whose pathway includes residential treatment, both initially and if there's a return to use, may face some confusing payment options. Public benefits (primarily Medicaid) vary from state to state. They're often insufficient for substance use treatment, especially for extended stays or long periods on medications. For years, federal statutes and some state laws have required health insurers to provide the same benefits for mental health/substance use issues as for physical health conditions, but these requirements didn't apply to all health insurance policies. Some states had more robust requirements and enforcement than others. The result was that access to care depended on whether you had "good insurance" and where you lived. Many people were left without coverage for addiction treatment. The federal Affordable Care

Act of 2010 changed some of that by identifying addiction treatment as an "essential service," which expanded coverage to millions of Americans.[28]

Unfortunately, the reality is that getting the right treatment paid for at the right time is rare. Families with health insurance continue to struggle to get insurance companies to pay for residential treatment. Some policies don't cover residential treatment for people under the age of eighteen. Others have a strict definition of "medical necessity" that can be a barrier. Some limit the number of treatment episodes per year. For some insurance companies, the first step is to deny a claim for addiction treatment and wait and see what happens. This can create delays at that critical time when people are ready to give treatment a try. Denied claims also can create huge financial commitments for families desperate to find treatment who decide to pay out-of-pocket and appeal the company's decision later. Parents I know have cashed in their full retirement to pay for their children's treatment, and others have spent months and years appealing denied claims.

Wellness

Andrew links the actions he takes to stay physically and emotionally healthy to the fundamental principles of his recovery. Andrew is in his mid-thirties and moved to Portland, Maine, after residential treatment in Massachusetts. He started taking college courses to complete a degree in chemistry he'd started years ago. During the first months of his recovery, Andrew was in bad shape from back surgeries and sports injuries, and he took small steps to wellness. "I started with the easy stuff, like drinking more water every day. Looking for water fountains on the university campus became a metaphor for me to look for ways to be healthy everywhere."

About two years into recovery, Andrew quit smoking. "That's one of the hardest things I've ever done. I swear it was harder to stop smoking than it was to quit using heroin."

Andrew worked on changing daily behaviors and set goals like showering and brushing and flossing his teeth every day. He created a consistent structure to his day, in contrast to the chaos of addiction. He went to the dentist, which he saw as a step toward greater accountability. "When you know you have a cavity, you make an appointment, and you act on it. That's accountability." Andrew has made a point of adopting good sleep habits, too. This can include having a regular sleep schedule, a ritual of winding down in a mindful way with meditation or yoga before sleep, and even spending money on a good mattress— all of which contribute to stress reduction and overall wellness.

Wellness is an essential aspect of recovery maintenance. Andrew's approach focused on the building blocks of good nutrition, physical activity, and good sleep habits. Healthy eating replenishes the body of depleted vitamins and minerals. Physical activity rebuilds lost muscle mass and elevates mood by recharging neurotransmitters like dopamine drained during drug use. Sleep repairs and restores the brain and body and contributes to energy and clear thinking the next day.

Nutrition

We don't know much about nutrition and malnutrition in people with addictions, even though they may have a genuine impact on the recovery process. In the early months of recovery, people may experience food cravings, especially for sweets, and depression related to nutrient deficiencies. They may have nutritional problems like mineral and vitamin deficiencies, metabolic disorders that compromise nutrition, and altered body composition (reduced body mass index) that go undetected.[29] People with a co-occurring eating disorder may find this part of wellness in recovery especially challenging.

Researchers have found that learning about good nutrition and following a new meal plan can aid a person's recovery journey—offering tools to improve nutrition in early recovery supports overall behavior change. Eating a balanced diet—proteins, grains, dairy, fruits, and vegetables—gives fresh fuel to the brain and body and promotes healing. For these reasons, starting with good nutrition in recovery is critical to overall wellness.[30] People in early recovery may want to have a nutritional assessment to create a food plan to restore the mineral balance. Setting small, manageable goals to change eating habits should be a part of an overall recovery plan. Learning to prepare food and cook meals can become a creative, relaxing, and social endeavor that lasts a lifetime.

Physical Activity

Researchers don't know much about the role of physical activity and exercise in the recovery process. Research hasn't yet confirmed the long-term benefits of physical activity when it comes to cravings, abstinence, and relapse, and researchers don't know how much exercise, what type of activity, and the intensity of exercise are best. They also don't know if it's best to work on endurance, strength, flexibility, balance, coordination, or some combination.[31, 32]

Even if research doesn't tell us much about physical activity and recovery, it makes sense to include some combination of aerobic exercise and strength training in a recovery plan to improve physical condition and reduce stress. Mind-body practices like yoga can help reduce pain, anxiety, and depression. It's probably a good idea to experiment with what works best at different stages of recovery. What is helpful in the early months of recovery might not be the same a few years down the road.

Sleep

It's essential to pay attention to sleep problems. Insomnia is about five times higher among people in early recovery than in the general population. Not getting enough sleep can create problems like low mood, being impulsive, and not regulating emotions. These are all triggers for a return to using.[33] For people who used alcohol or drugs to fall asleep, removing them can make nighttime difficult. Using sleeping pills is usually not an option. Habits that create healthy sleep are the same for people in recovery as everyone else. Limiting naps, reducing caffeine consumption, going to bed and getting up at the same time every day, and sleeping seven or eight hours every night are essential. Making sure to get enough exposure to sunlight, avoiding heavy meals at night, getting exercise during the day, creating a relaxing space to sleep in, and establishing a bedtime routine are good ideas as well. Sleep that isn't drug-induced is one of the many gifts of recovery.

Stress

Negative emotions like anger and stressful situations can trigger using again. In addition to one-on-one counseling, support groups, exercise, mindfulness practices, and yoga can be effective stress-reducing tools in treatment and recovery.[34, 35]

Abstinence

Recovery isn't the same as abstinence, but they frequently go together. For some people in recovery, abstaining from any mind-altering substance is essential for maintaining health and wellness. If they're using drugs or alcohol, they're less likely to maintain a daily routine, eat and sleep right, and seek regular health care. For others, moderate use of alcohol or drugs like cannabis doesn't get in the way of a healthy lifestyle.

What Can Allies Do?

For Family Members

- Support tobacco cessation when your loved one is ready to quit. While the focus needs to be on supporting our family member's chosen recovery path, we shouldn't forget tobacco cessation. Help your loved one by asking them if it's OK for you to help them find free tobacco-cessation resources in your state. This usually includes free telephone "quit lines" and online support. Many states have free nicotine replacement patches for people who are income eligible. We can also help by suggesting they check their insurance policy to see what it covers and encouraging a conversation with a primary care physician about quitting.

- Don't make assumptions about health consequences. Old ideas about who gets cirrhosis of the liver (only old men who drank their entire lives) are not accurate. Alcohol use has increased considerably in the past twenty years in people of all ages and ethnic groups. The consequences—especially liver disease—have increased most dramatically in people in their twenties and thirties, and health care providers have been astounded at the number of young people with advanced liver disease.[36]

- Ask your loved one if they would like you to make a doctor's appointment and go with them to the doctor's office. The tasks of everyday living, in addition to lining up counseling appointments, job interviews, or childcare arrangements, can feel overwhelming in early recovery, and it might be easy to skip adding a doctor's appointment to the to-do list. By making the call and being present at the appointment (if that's what they want), we can help lessen feelings of shame, and we can make sure the doctor is not adding to it by using stigmatizing language or discouraging talk. We also can help by going to the pharmacy to pick up any prescription medications after the appointment. These may seem like simple actions, but for people who are managing a lot of changes in their lives and who may have had some bad experiences in hospitals, doctors' offices, and pharmacies, it can be reassuring to have help and support.

- Ask your loved one if they would like you to make an appointment with a dentist. They might not have practiced good dental hygiene for many years, and oral health problems might have mounted up. Taking care of cavities and other oral health issues is vital for overall health. It's also important because untreated dental pain needs to be managed so that they don't seek painkillers. If your loved one is in recovery from opioid addiction, be sure to mention this if dental work requires pain relief afterward.

- Ask your loved one if they would like you to help with insurance details. If your loved one takes you up on the offer and has insurance, you can help wade through the muddle of prior authorizations, co-pays, and deductibles to make sure they get the care they need. If they don't have insurance, you can help look for public options or free care.

  Questions you can ask the insurance company include:

  - What level of care does this plan support? Detox? Residential treatment? For how long? What about care after treatment?

  - Does treatment require prior authorization, preapproval, or a referral?

  - What are the co-pays involved?

  - What is the maximum out-of-pocket expense?

  - Which treatment providers in my area are covered?

For Community Organizations

- Reach out to local recovery groups and offer healthy eating and cooking classes, exercise classes, etc.

- Offer "recovery yoga" or "trauma-sensitive yoga" and other forms of holistic healing specifically for people in recovery.
- Work with local recovery groups to offer recovery retreats at local venues.

For Employers

- Include people in recovery on workplace wellness committees.
- Check the health insurance benefits you provide employees to be sure substance use treatment (including multiple rounds of treatment) is reimbursed at a reasonable rate for employees and their family members. Make sure employees know about their benefits.
- Find ways to incentivize healthy eating and physical activity through health insurance, free workplace programs, and free gym memberships.
- Offer healthy eating and cooking classes.

For Health Care Providers

- Make a point of offering smoking cessation services to your patients in recovery.
- Consider implementing recovery management checkups, similar to ongoing monitoring of other chronic health conditions like diabetes.
- Ask your patients in recovery if they would like a referral for a nutrition assessment.

13

SPIRITUAL HEALTH

"I JUST GET goosebumps when you ask about my lasting recovery," Sarah says, *"because it just never ceases to amaze me that life is the way that it is today. It's not perfect. There are still plenty of struggles, and that familiar restlessness crops up at times. So, it's not that it's just completely gone, but I'm so familiar with it at this point that it just doesn't consume me the way that it used to. And I have a degree of peace and comfort inside myself that I just never, ever, ever, ever would have thought could have been possible for somebody like me.*

"I connect with this miraculous feeling about my recovery. It's a miracle! It's a miracle I'm alive! It's a miracle that we're alive! I have a very rich spiritual life that has taken me in this circle from looking for something outside myself through the spiritual lens, like it's going to be some practice or some teacher or some book that's going to help me. And it's been this big circle, like searching, searching, searching, searching, and I would just come back to where I am in any given moment, like washing the dishes or mopping the floor or whatever it is. There's a sacredness in every moment, and I work on living from that sacredness as much as possible.

"The beauty of recovery never ceases to amaze me. When I think about it deeply, I can go pretty quickly to the core of existence. Like I'm standing there doing the dishes thinking, 'This is life with a capital L.' It's wonderful. I can get there really, really fast. There's so much to be in awe of. One of the biggest gifts of my recovery is being able to connect to that inspiring experience of just being alive."

Sarah's spiritual reflection is like many stories of people in recovery who have found a richness in daily living and are grateful simply to be alive. Being in recovery from addiction isn't the only way to find that fullness, and not all people in recovery experience it. But recovery can help create it.

A recurring theme in my interviews with people in recovery is the healing power of love and connection. Trauma, broken relationships, and the jagged life that arises from addiction create painful scars. Those in the recovery community have experienced the untimely deaths of far too many family members, friends, and colleagues to overdose. Some come from toxic families of origin or have burned all bridges with their family members. Many find it helpful to call on love and connection to each other and the universe to help understand their lives in addiction, repair their broken relationships (including with God or another higher power), forgive and accept themselves and each other, and move their lives forward in a spiritually healthy way.

Niki grew up with nonpracticing Catholic parents in a tiny town in northern Maine. Growing up, she stayed away from God. "If He existed, He wouldn't have permitted the things that happened to me as a kid. I thought I'd go to hell for all of the things I did anyway."

Then, in her forties and after years of substance use, she went to a residential treatment facility for women. Some of the women invited her to The Lost Coin, a church in Portland, Maine, in a building that used to be a bar. "I was so excited about my recovery," she says, "I was up for anything, and so I went. There was a street party there with a band, and I loved music, so everything just fit—new life, party in the street, music, in a 'redeemed bar'—God met me where I needed to be.

"Where does our knowledge about doing the right thing come from?" Niki asks. "We're taught, there are laws, and there is some stuff we just know. So, I know when I'm doing something wrong. I spent a lifetime going against that inner knowing of right and wrong. I was living with a disconnect. I wanted to stop hurting people, but I just didn't know how to stop. Everything I had tried to do right by myself, I kept messing it up. I felt condemned to hell. I was condemning me. I was beating me down."

Niki's path included 12-step meetings, and there, people simplified things for her, saying, "'You know what the wrong thing is. If you don't know what the right thing is, don't do anything at all. Ask someone.' That was very simple and practical."

Niki's faith came from wanting to do the "next right thing," an often-heard piece of advice in AA. That was the beginning of really being able to apply the idea of faith, talking to God about it, learning to trust. "I don't have to be perfect, and I'm not in charge. For me, in recovery, at first, I wanted to fix everything—I wanted to fix myself—I thought everything has to be good all the time. Now faith gives me space to allow things to be as they are. It also allows me to know where my part is in that. I am part of life, but I am not in charge of life.

"I'm in conversation with God all the time—in moments when things are going well, 'Thank you'; when I'm struggling, I can sit still and wait until I feel the next right thing. Faith is an action, not a thing. I remind myself that I have a small part in a big play. Life isn't all about me, and I have to be right-sized. I am not God. This is a practical, realistic view of life.

"Faith helps me know there are times when I need to do things about life and times when I just have to let go. I learned this in recovery, and now it's the space I go to for everything. I feel like faith is my breath. Without it, I'm a mess, trying to manipulate and control, and I miss all of my right-now moments. Faith is my life force. Without it, I can't live."

Paths to Spiritual Wellness

12-Step Programs

Acceptance of a higher power and experiencing a spiritual awakening are at the core of 12-step programs, including Alcoholics Anonymous. Because AA has been the mainstay of recovery in the United States since it began in Ohio in 1935, this language is familiar to most of us. People in 12-step programs find a fount of support in their higher power and turn their lives over to it and the wisdom of a like-minded group of fellow recovering adults. AA's path toward a spiritual awakening also includes helping others, which creates a meaningful and sometimes sacred connection that may have powerful healing effects.

Many people in AA connect with the God of Christianity. That connection may be unacceptable to atheists, agnostics, and non-Christians, as well as to those who have experienced harm and judgment in Christian churches. Still, many who don't believe in the Christian God, or any god, find AA helpful in their recovery.[1] They may consider their higher power to be the presence of helpful others, the human experience, nature, goodness, or, simply, love.[2] The 12 steps have been modified to incorporate Buddhism, Islam, Judaism, and other religious beliefs and spiritual practices.[3]

Recovery Ministries

Some Christian churches place recovery from addiction at the center of their ministry. They reach out to people who are actively using as well as people in recovery and offer food, clothing, peer support, and Christian fellowship. Others offer Celebrate Recovery, a biblical program for people in recovery, and Christ-centered 12-step meetings as well as opportunities to volunteer and be part of a large Christian family. In the Black communities, churches can be especially supportive of recovery. As one Black man said, "In our [Black] community, recovery doesn't look like going to AA meetings. Sometimes it looks like going to church."

Wellbriety

Wellbriety is a blending of the 12-step path with Native American traditions and practices of healing, such as the medicine wheel (which encompasses dimensions of health and the cycle of life) and talking circles (a traditional way of solving problems that involves everyone in the community equally).

Buddhism and Mindfulness Meditation

Some people who commit to a Buddhist path and practice acknowledge the Four Noble Truths and apply them to addiction and recovery: (1) Wanting and craving (addiction) are the cause of suffering; (2) We suffer because we insist that we can satisfy our cravings; (3) It's possible to end the suffering (the emotional underpinnings of wanting and craving); and (4) The way to end suffering is through a way of life that follows the Eightfold Path of wise understanding, intention, speech, action, livelihood, effort, mindfulness, and concentration.[4] This path includes daily meditation practices, investigations into the causes and conditions of addiction, and ways to find or create a healing community.

Mindfulness meditation is a Buddhist practice to unify the body and mind as a path to enhanced spiritual well-being. Mindfulness meditation has entered mainstream culture, including people in recovery, and evidence suggests that it is as effective as other interventions as a way to reduce stress and anxiety and address depression by quieting the mind and increasing focus.[5] Many people in recovery practice yoga, which may be similarly effective in reducing stress and anxiety.[6]

Research

Spirituality plays a significant role in recovery for some people, and for others, it doesn't matter much. Some turn to organized religion; some return to the faith of their childhood. Other people find mindfulness meditation is helpful without a spiritual component. Experiences vary considerably across age, gender, ethnicity, culture, and race, and it's difficult to make any definitive statements about spirituality or religion. Generally, they appear to be more important among Black people than white people and Hispanic people, and women generally find spirituality and faith more important for overcoming problems than men. People who attend formal treatment or 12-step meetings are more likely to identify spirituality as an important part of their recovery than people who don't.[7]

For something that is so fundamental to recovery for some people—spiritual practice—it's surprising that there's very little research to back up its importance. Scientific research on the role of spirituality and religion in recovery is in its infancy. There's very little evidence for how or why they're helpful in recovery.[8, 9, 10] Even in 12-step programs with a solid spiritual base, the spiritual "mechanisms" explain only a small part of their effectiveness.[11, 12]

What Can Allies Do?

For Everyone

- Be curious. Find out more. Do the work needed to become open-hearted. As Niki said, "When we feel judged, and we're trying to grow, are you growing too? Come back to a place of love and empathy with us." Another man said, "Be willing to sacrifice. Give up your old beliefs about people with addiction and learn a new, loving way."

For Faith-Based Organizations

- Ask members of your congregation who are in recovery how to create a recovery-friendly place of worship and meditation and then work together to make that happen.

- Reach out to local recovery groups and invite people in recovery to join worship services, church meals, community volunteer days, and other social gatherings.

- Share your faith with people who are struggling with drug or alcohol problems. Ask how you can help by simply saying, "How can I help?"

For Yoga Instructors and Mindfulness Meditation Practitioners

- Learn about recovery yoga, meditation, and trauma-sensitive yoga. Consider offering a class. Reach out to a local recovery community center to offer a free class there.

14

MEDICATIONS FOR ADDICTION[1]

SARAH SIEGEL HAS a great life. She has a family, and she's a recovery coach and a spiritual leader. She loves to meditate, read about different religious paths, play with her dogs, and grow her own food. But her life hasn't always been like this. About fifteen years ago, when Sarah was addicted to heroin, a doctor told her that she would die if she kept using it. "I always felt like death was just there every second, looking over my shoulder," Sarah said about that time, and she decided to go on methadone. "I feel like choosing methadone really was that decision to pick life from a place that I didn't have much to hold on to. And so, for me, deciding to go to the methadone clinic was really about choosing life, deciding that I wanted to live."

Sarah's story isn't unusual for people with opioid addiction. Brushes with death and feeling desperate about how to get out of the life of addiction create a depressing downward spiral that's hard to stop. Her recovery journey included medication that formed the foundation to rebuild her life in the first years of recovery. "I worked hard, really hard," she says. "And I couldn't have done that without methadone, but ultimately, it was through all of that hard work that I found lasting recovery."

For centuries, researchers, health care providers, and charlatans have been hunting for a tonic or medication to treat or cure addiction.[2] These days, some people turn to health care providers for prescription drugs, and others experiment with plant-based treatments for opioid addiction. The Food and Drug Administration (FDA) has approved therapies for the medical management of opioid use disorder. People in recovery have developed their own practices with drugs like cannabis, kratom, ibogaine, ketamine, and psilocybin. This chapter focuses on FDA-approved medications.

A NOTE ON LANGUAGE

It's hard to keep pace with the changing terminology for treatments for opioid addiction. The terms methadone maintenance, opioid replacement (or substitution) therapy, and medication-assisted treatment (MAT) have fallen out of favor in health care circles. Even so, MAT is the most common way to talk about medications for opioid addiction in the recovery community. Beyond that realm, the current thinking is to call methadone, the various formulations of buprenorphine (Suboxone), and naltrexone medications for opioid use disorder (MOUD), medications for addiction (MFA), or simply pharmacotherapy.[3] Some consider these medications as part of recovery and refer to them as medication-assisted recovery (MAR).[4] Still others see medications for opioid addiction as harm reduction, keeping people alive until they seek residential or outpatient treatment, or until their recovery is based on abstinence.

Medications for Opioid Use Disorder

The FDA has approved methadone, buprenorphine, buprenorphine plus naloxone, and naltrexone for the medical management of opioid use disorder.[5] Generally, in the recovery, treatment, and health care communities, all formulations of buprenorphine are referred to by the trade name Suboxone, which will be used in this book. Naltrexone isn't yet widely used and won't be discussed here.

People who have opioid use disorder experience intense withdrawal symptoms and powerful cravings when they stop using opioids. Withdrawal from opioids is unlike withdrawal from other substances like alcohol or cannabis. It can be so hard that they just want it to stop, and the only way to do that is by taking more opioids. Medications for addiction calm the withdrawal symptoms and reduce cravings so people can get on with their lives. The evidence is clear that these medications reduce the risk of overdose more than treatment without them.[6] For some people, these drugs are lifesavers in a literal way—preventing overdose—and symbolically, because they give people a chance to put their lives back together. "It saved my life" is a common refrain in discussions about Suboxone.

Methadone

Methadone is an opioid prescribed to relieve the cravings and withdrawal effects experienced in recovery. It replaces other opioids a person may be using. Since 1972 when the FDA approved it as a medication for heroin addiction, it has been heavily regulated in the United States. People using it as part of their recovery are required to go to special clinics, sometimes daily, to receive their liquid dose. (Prescription methadone for pain is in pill form and may be prescribed by health care providers with an appropriate license from the federal Drug Enforcement Agency.) This system of methadone clinics creates enormous inconveniences that can be barriers to recovery. One man I know who lived in a rural part of Maine got up at 5 a.m. every day to drive to the clinic, ninety miles away, to get his methadone. Then he went back to his hometown to start work at 8 a.m. He was in his thirties, married, with two young children, and without the strong support of his family and employer, it would have been challenging to keep that schedule and maintain his recovery. Despite his many efforts, he wasn't permitted to receive take-home doses but continued this schedule for the first several years of his recovery.

Suboxone

Before the FDA approved Suboxone in 2002, health care providers, policy makers, and scientists viewed treating opioid addiction with methadone as the "gold standard" of care. Today, it's Suboxone, which trained primary care providers can prescribe as part of overall patient care, with weekly or monthly prescriptions. In 2000, Congress established training requirements for physicians to prescribe Suboxone and further required them to provide patients with counseling or refer them to counseling services. As the overdose crisis deepened, advocates in the recovery community and others viewed the eight-hour training requirement and counseling as significant barriers to care. In 2021, the US Department of Health and Human Services (HHS) issued new guidelines that permitted physicians, physician assistants, nurse practitioners, clinical nurse specialists, certified registered nurse anesthetists, and certified nurse midwives an exemption from these requirements.[7]

Both methadone and Suboxone are considered evidence-based treatments for opioid addiction, including for pregnant women, and neither one is "better" than the other. Many people prefer Suboxone because it is more widely available and doesn't require daily trips to a special clinic. Others don't find that Suboxone successfully reduces cravings and take methadone instead. Both medications themselves are opioids and are federally controlled substances, and they may be diverted to illegal use and used to get high.[8] Health care providers believe these risks are minimized when these medications are appropriately prescribed and taken as directed. Some people in the recovery community think otherwise. Suboxone is readily available on the streets and in jails and prisons, sometimes used to get high but more often used to mitigate withdrawal symptoms in people who don't or can't get it legally. Most times, people seeing a doctor for a prescription have already tried it and may even know the dose that works best for reducing their cravings when they arrive at the doctor's office for the first time. ·

Medically Supervised Withdrawal and Treatment

Medically supervised withdrawal and treatment facilities use Suboxone to help patients manage the symptoms of opioid withdrawal, like muscle aches, restlessness, anxiety, runny nose, inability to sleep, excessive sweating, diarrhea, nausea, vomiting, and high blood pressure. Symptoms usually lessen in seventy-two hours or so, and after a week, many are gone altogether. When patients are stable, the best course of action is to go to appropriate treatment. If that's not available, they go home or back to the streets.

Overdose

Medications for opioid use disorder help people stay alive. The most common times for opioid overdose are after a person hasn't been using opioids for a while, like after leaving treatment or jail or prison. During that time—a day, a week, or a month—tolerance for the drug decreases, and the body needs less to obtain the same effect. If the drug cravings are intense and people start using again, they might use too much, shutting down their central nervous system and leading to an overdose. This risk for overdose death sets opioid addiction apart from other addictions—stopping use without medications is dangerous and can lead to relapse, overdose, and sometimes death. In this regard, abstinence can be a pathway to death.

Stigma

People from all walks of life take medications for opioid use disorder. They have jobs and families and want to be contributing members of the community. They are business owners, teachers, nurses, lawyers, and come from just about every profession or field. Even so, they face harsh judgment almost everywhere in the community. They experience prejudice and discrimination among substance use counselors and their peers in recovery who prefer abstinence, pharmacies where they pick up their prescription, health care providers treating other conditions, staff at medical practices, and neighbors who see them going in and out of a methadone clinic. For people on long-term methadone therapy, the stigma and feelings of shame can go on for years or even decades. The tensions are palpable between people who promote an abstinence-only approach and those who support medications as a vital part of recovery. So far, no amount of education for people in recovery, health care providers, and community members has managed to calm these conflicts. It's no wonder people typically aren't public about medication being part of their recovery.

New Models for Addiction Treatment

Health care providers and policy makers are looking at new ways to increase access to medications for opioid addiction, especially Suboxone. The federal government has launched numerous grant-funded initiatives and pumped millions of dollars into programs to encourage states and health care systems to train primary care providers and encourage them to prescribe Suboxone. Integrating substance use counseling into primary care settings where Suboxone is prescribed is one way.[9] Another is initiating Suboxone treatment for emergency room patients, linking them to a recovery coach, and providing a referral to a primary care provider for follow-up care. Research shows that if people who are using opioids receive Suboxone as part of an emergency room visit, they are more likely to engage in some form of substance use treatment and use fewer illegal opioids afterward.[10]

Some recovery community centers include Suboxone prescribing on site so that people have direct links to recovery peer support and opportunities to increase their recovery capital the moment treatment begins. The jury is still out as to whether this is an effective way to increase access to medications.

The Role of Big Pharma

People in recovery from opioid addiction whom I have talked with have strong opinions about pharmaceutical companies and generally lump them together as "Big Pharma," even though many are not involved in the production of opioids. "They're responsible for the opioid crisis, no doubt," said one person. "Killers!" said another. "They should pay for what they've done," said a third. Even though some benefited from lifesaving medications, including methadone, Suboxone, and naloxone, they felt the long arm of Big Pharma pushing prescription painkillers onto them and their friends for years. That pushing, they think, continues with Suboxone. There's money to be made in addiction medications, and federal policies support Suboxone as a "blockbuster drug." Big Pharma has shown up on both sides—pushing addictive opioids first and then supplying remedies for opioid addiction a few years later—and it's easy to understand why recovery advocates have rallied around class-action suits against pharmaceutical companies for their unscrupulous marketing practices for opioids.

Medications and Recovery

Danielle Rideout is the recovery liaison for four small police departments in rural Maine. She serves as a case manager for people with substance use disorder and helps them get connected with services. She listens to their stories, cheers them on, and shares their joys and sorrows. Getting to this point in her life wasn't easy. Danielle has been in recovery for almost fourteen years. Her recovery path included taking Suboxone, participating in a support group for mothers, volunteering in her community, and attending 12-step meetings. She had a whole lot of family and community support, too.

Danielle took Suboxone for six and a half years, and she credits it for the things she's been able to do in her recovery. "I'm a Licensed Alcohol and Drug Counselor. I'm going to grad school. I own a house, and I have two children. I'm married to the man I've been with for fifteen years. We have all of these things, and they're all a direct result of my recovery. I truly believe Suboxone did that for me," she says.

For Danielle, Suboxone was only part of her recovery. "It wasn't like I was just using Suboxone for my recovery. There were other things, too," she says. Being part of the moms' support group, going to meetings, volunteering, reconnecting with her community, and going back to school were important, too.

Talking about stigma, Danielle says, "Everybody is different. It doesn't matter if someone can get sober and stay sober without Suboxone. That's great, but that's not my story, and that's not how it worked for me. Recovery is a process. We have to go through everything we've gone through to get to where we are today."

Researchers have flooded journals with articles about Suboxone, including how long a person should continue taking it. Opinions differ, with no consensus. Most patients discontinue it within a few weeks or months, even though treatment outcomes (measured in emergency room visits, hospitalizations, and drug overdoses) begin to improve after at least fifteen months of taking it.[11] Some, like Danielle, take it for several years. Many people I talked with benefited from combining Suboxone with attending 12-step programs. Evidence shows that attending 12-step meetings doesn't seem to interfere with Suboxone treatment and may actually result in better outcomes.[12]

Not everyone has a good experience taking methadone or Suboxone. They may be the "gold standard" for treatment of opioid use disorder, but they aren't a silver bullet. Many people taking medications have little in the way of recovery support or recovery capital, making sustained recovery challenging. Some people don't like how the medications make them feel, and they work hard to taper off them as soon as possible. (Both have possible side effects that include constipation, diarrhea, headache, and nausea.) People I talked with who had taken Suboxone said they felt emotionally "flat" while on it. Some who used Suboxone or methadone to get high at one point don't want anything to do with them as part of their recovery. Drug dealers prowl in the parking lot of some poorly operated methadone clinics, making it tough to believe it's actual treatment. Many of the people I interviewed admitted to getting drugs at or near the clinic where they got their methadone. For

Suboxone, in particular, many people who have been treated poorly by health care providers are unimpressed with yet another doctor with a prescription pad and not enough other support to help them get well.

As Suboxone has become widely available, health care providers and treatment agencies have looked for ways to create easy access to it, sometimes without creating links to adequate recovery support services, including housing. Some people believe that sending a person who is experiencing homelessness back to the streets with a Suboxone prescription and no safe housing is a prescription for disaster and even death. This reflects a tension between people who see the urgent need for Suboxone to save lives no matter what and others who consider the focus on this drug as diminishing the meaning of recovery to a physical problem and shortchanging people from true wellness. Some recovery advocates feel that health care providers readily toss "bupe" at people with opioid addiction without any additional support. It's a "quick fix" that doesn't fix anything. They see their friends in active opioid use become part of an endless churn of overdosing, going to an emergency room, getting Suboxone and a referral to a primary care doctor but no recovery support services, hitting the streets again, and starting all over. Or their friends have the best intentions in treatment, take a Suboxone prescription, and head out the door without sufficient recovery supports to help create a good life, relapse, and start all over again.

Medications for Opioid Use Disorder and Pregnancy

Pregnant women with opioid use disorder may also be on methadone or Subutex, the buprenorphine formulation for pregnant women. (Most people refer to this as Suboxone, too.) In fact, they're first in line for treatment because opioid addiction creates a significant risk to the baby's health. Withdrawal can bring on a miscarriage or early delivery, and medications for addiction can prevent that. Unfortunately, as with other forms of addiction treatment, access to Subutex is hopelessly inadequate in many parts of the country. And women of color are less likely to receive medications during pregnancy than white women.[13]

Being pregnant can motivate women to seek treatment and sustain their recovery. One study showed that women who can access Subutex early in pregnancy are more likely to remain in treatment a year after they give birth.[14] And yet, pregnant women on methadone or Subutex face powerful stigma. "Women are more stigmatized than men," Honesty, a woman who used drugs during her pregnancy nineteen years ago, told me. "We're supposed to make babies, not use drugs." She was mandated to take methadone after the birth to keep her child, but what helped her the most was living in a recovery residence with other women with the same problem. "The women who went before me showed me the way," she explained. She's been in recovery for more than fifteen years, and her daughter—the baby she carried while she was using heroin—is healthy, happy, and ready to graduate from high school.

Danielle and Sarah were on addiction medications during their pregnancies. Deciding to go on methadone was hard for Sarah. "For me, it was a forced acceptance that I was actually sick enough in my addiction that I couldn't just pull myself out of it." It didn't help that she felt judgment all around her. "When I walked into the doctor's office, there was just this assumption that I didn't care about my child, and that wasn't true. For the first time in my life, I think I felt a sense of purpose that I had never experienced before. I felt just in awe that there was a being growing inside of me, and I had this drive to really care for myself in a different way. Everything that I did was so centered on the fact that I was pregnant, and I couldn't wait to meet my child."

What Can Allies Do?

For Everyone

- Learn about medications for addiction and where they are prescribed in your community. The Substance Abuse and Mental Health Services Administration's website provides a good overview of medications to treat addiction: www.samhsa.gov/medication-assisted-treatment.

- Examine your attitudes toward medications for addiction compared with medications for other conditions.

- Try to use nonstigmatizing language about medications as part of the recovery process.

For Family Members

- If someone in your family is taking medication for addiction, ask if they are open to talking about it, and find out what it's like for them. If they're also in counseling, ask if there is anything they want you to do to support that. If they're going to a recovery community center, ask if you can go, too, to see what it's like and show your support for their recovery.

- If they're taking methadone, ask them if you can help them with regular transportation for daily or weekly doses. If they have take-home doses, ask if you can help them keep the doses safe from children and anyone who might be tempted to use it to get high.

For Health Care Providers

- Spend some time talking with people in recovery. Journal articles that describe the medical aspects of prescribing medications don't typically discuss recovery—that self-directed process of change toward wellness—and talking with your patients in recovery is one of the best ways to learn.

- Visit recovery residences where medications for addiction are allowed and learn what requirements the residences have to store and dispense medications.

- If you're a Suboxone prescriber, talk to your peers about what it's like and why you chose to incorporate that into your practice.

- Attend and participate in a town hall and other community meetings about addiction and recovery, and be ready to talk about addiction medications to dispel myths and misperceptions. Tell stories about your patients on Suboxone who have been able to work and enjoy their family life.

- If you're part of a program to provide easy access to Suboxone in emergency rooms, try spending some time with the people you treat to find out how it's working for them. If you're seeing the same patients repeatedly, maybe it's time to make some changes in the program so they have more recovery support when you discharge them.

SECTION 5
The Pillars of Recovery:
Home

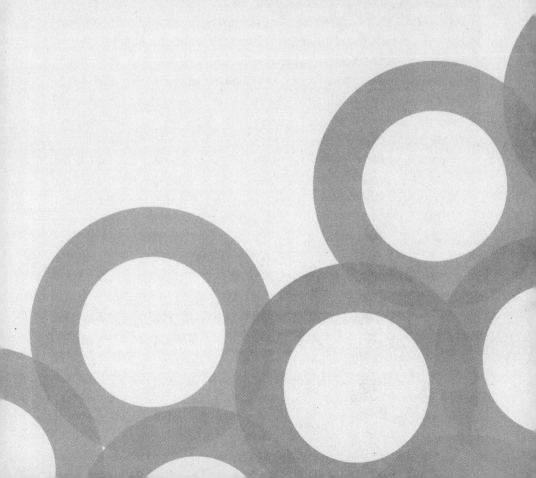

15

RECOVERY HOUSING[1]

ANDREW IS IN long-term recovery and works as a chemist for a private firm that produces plastic coatings in Massachusetts. Before that, though, he had a severe problem with drugs and alcohol. His drinking started in his teens, and in his twenties, a physician prescribed opioids for pain after back surgery. The physician abruptly stopped the prescription, leaving Andrew in withdrawal and seeking relief, and he eventually turned to heroin. By the time he was in his early thirties, his drug use was peppered with short periods of recovery, and he'd been in and out of residential treatment and lived in several recovery residences in Maine and Massachusetts.

"Living with peers was important," Andrew tells me, as he describes the first few months of life in a recovery residence. "They understood the recovery process, and they had compassion." He formed strong and deep bonds with the men in the recovery residences. "The people you live with understand you, help you feel the most connected, push and challenge you all at the same time."

The structure of the recovery residence was important, too. "I created a framework of accountability in the house for how to live in recovery after I moved out," Andrew explains. After years of focusing on getting high and using drugs, he had a lot to learn about managing his personal life and relationships in a healthy way. The recovery residence rules created "a great deal of accountability," which he internalized, and which inform his life now. He also learned how to develop relationships based on mutual respect and trust. "The recovery residence was a good place to practice having a stable home, with many personalities and issues that came up. We all had to figure out how to live together peacefully."

After dropping out of college in his twenties, Andrew returned to college while living in the recovery residence. He started with one course at the University of Southern Maine. "I was afraid to walk on campus alone," he says. "I didn't know how to be a student and be sober." But the support he received from the men in his recovery residence gave him the confidence to show up to class every day. He graduated with a degree in chemistry.

When Andrew was ready to live on his own, he found an apartment in downtown Portland, where he could live without a car and walk to campus. The landlord asked for the first and last month's rent, plus a security deposit, plus six months' rent, for a total of nine months' rent. His family came up with the nearly $10,000 required upfront for him to live independently. "I was lucky," Andrew says. "My family had resources to support me in the recovery residence and afterward, too. Not everyone is so fortunate."

Many people enter recovery at home, and as family members, we learn alongside them how to live this new life in wellness. We do our best to change our own behaviors to support them and stay healthy ourselves. But living at home isn't always possible or even desirable. Some people have burned all their bridges, including with family members. Others, like Andrew, need to get on to the next stage of their lives and independent living. Still others have no home or family to return to. In these situations, going to a recovery residence—what used to be called a sober house, sober living, or a halfway house—is an important option.[2]

According to David Sheridan, executive director of the National Alliance for Recovery Residences, an organization committed to improving access to quality recovery residences, the recovery residences of today grew out of an informal word-of-mouth network developed in the 12-step community years ago.[3] People would go to 12-step meetings and find out about people they could live with if they had no place else to go. Often this was "hit or miss" in terms of quality or finding a house that was a good fit. Now that's changing. People can still connect at 12-step meetings with people who will give them a place to sleep, but more formal recovery residences are springing up in cities, towns, and a few rural areas to provide safe housing for people in early recovery.

As Andrew learned, a recovery residence can be an excellent place for a new start. This chapter explores how to find quality recovery housing, some pitfalls, and what communities can do to support recovery residences.

Safe Housing

Safe housing for people in recovery means more than living in a place that has passed building, fire, and safety code inspections or in a neighborhood with low crime rates. These things may ensure physical safety but don't necessarily foster wellness or personal and spiritual growth. Safe housing is the foundation for healthy relationships and healthy living in recovery. It's a secure place for self-exploration, a place to learn new behaviors and attitudes, experiment with new ways of living, and build recovery capital. In other words, safe housing is a home.

Preventing relapse and safe housing are closely linked. Most treatment includes developing a relapse-prevention plan. Counselors help clients identify triggers—situations where there's a high risk of drinking or drugging again—and develop healthy strategies to cope. Triggers in early recovery include physical withdrawal symptoms and cravings for drugs or alcohol, being with people using drugs, being where you used to buy drugs, or being around drug paraphernalia like needles, bottles of liquor, or bongs. Triggers can also be internal experiences, like feeling anger or sadness in personal relationships or worrying about money. Lack of sleep, isolation, and stressful life events are common triggers for relapse.[4]

Having a safe place to live in early recovery means being in a place where relapse prevention and relapse resilience (staying healthy after a relapse) are priorities. That means staying away from the people and places where drug use occurred; building new social networks of people who don't use drugs or alcohol; developing healthy eating, exercise, and sleeping habits; avoiding stressful situations, including difficult personal relationships; and learning how to cope with difficult emotions. In addition, research shows that people with strong social support are less likely to relapse, so a safe place to live also includes strong peer support from fellow housemates.[5]

Recovery Residences

Ron is a retired physician in his sixties. After he completed medical school and was working for a small clinic in Alaska, Ron's substance use interfered with his work. He sought treatment at the Betty Ford Center in Rancho Mirage, California. After five weeks, he was referred to a recovery residence in Yakima, Washington, where he lived for two months. He became a staff member and continued to live there for another six months, providing services and support to the residents.

Fast-forward to 2014, and Ron again lived in a recovery residence, this time in Portland, Maine, following a relapse and another stint in residential treatment. When I ask him about his housing experiences, he emphasizes that he always "had a place to stay or a home to go back to." Like most physicians in recovery, he had a significant amount of recovery capital in the form of education, housing, transportation, and financial assets, all of which contributed significantly to his recovery. "Both [recovery] houses gave me an opportunity to make a new start ... under the guidance of people who have demonstrated success in recovery." In addition, staff at the houses provided basic needs and structure, both of which were missing at times during his active use, and that allowed him the time and energy to focus on living free of harmful substances and experiencing "a contented sobriety."

Recovery houses provide peer support, structure, accountability, and physical safety that people need in early recovery. Houses can be owned by an individual and run by a house manager (often a former house resident). Some treatment agencies operate recovery houses as part of the agency's continuum of care for patients. Nonprofit organizations and religious groups also run houses. In some areas, real estate investors are working with property management companies to create recovery housing options.

Recovery residences run on the "social model" of recovery that understands recovery as an interaction between the individual in recovery and the environment. For recovery residences, the environment in the house is as close to a safe home life as possible, based on local community norms. The social model approach shifts the emphasis of solutions for alcohol and drug problems from the individual to the community of peers for recovery support, creating accountability by involving house residents in chores, decision making, conflict resolution, and governance, and using personal recovery experiences to help others.[6] Each resident agrees to create and follow a personalized recovery plan and abide by house rules that foster a recovery-friendly environment.

Using the social model of recovery creates opportunities for different recovery residences based on religion and spirituality, sexual orientation, gender identification, and cultural and socioeconomic backgrounds. Residences come in all shapes and sizes, and monthly fees vary. Low-cost houses offer little in the way of programs or services, and some recovery residences are no more than a rented apartment with subleases for each bedroom. More expensive residences provide various services, including help with job hunting, transportation, gourmet food, health club memberships, and treatment-oriented programs on site.

Most recovery residences are single-sex, and some houses allow parents in recovery to live with their small children. Peer support in recovery residences tends to be informal through support groups and day-to-day interactions with fellow housemates. Residents are expected to give support to their housemates, not just receive it. Some places include trained recovery coaches. Most house managers receive some level of training in peer recovery support and serve as recovery role models for residents. Many houses plan social outings, shared meals, and celebrations of residents' milestones (like getting a job) to build relationships. Nearly all recovery residences require abstinence from mind-altering substances. A handful practice harm reduction and allow, for example, cannabis on site. A growing number of houses accept residents who are on medications for addiction.

While most people live in a recovery residence immediately after substance use treatment, hospitalization, or incarceration, some choose to live in sober-living environments without going to treatment. This choice may be for financial reasons—no access to health care coverage to pay for treatment—or because of a disagreement with the way residential treatment facilities operate. Some people prefer to approach sober living and recovery on their own terms rather than on terms laid out by counselors and treatment agencies.

Research

Research on recovery housing as a recovery support service is positive, and research is underway to deepen our knowledge of exactly what about recovery residences is most helpful.[7] Research to date shows that people in residential treatment are more successful if they have recovery support services, including safe housing, after they complete treatment. Most people who live in recovery residences reduce or eliminate their drug use while in the house, and many maintain abstinence after leaving.[8, 9] It may come as a surprise that recovery residences create an economic benefit to communities compared with the cost of doing nothing. One study showed a cost savings of $29,000 per person compared with returning to the community without this recovery support. Cost savings were predominantly from reduced illegal activity.[10] Research also shows that recovery residences add to the quality of life in a neighborhood because residents often help neighbors with chores and participate in local community events.[11]

Quality Control

Until recently, local and state governments and the federal government paid little attention to recovery housing. Because the houses are considered single-family residences rather than treatment facilities, state laws and licensing requirements don't apply. Few operating standards and protections were in place for residents. Nationwide, the rapid increase in the number of recovery residences in response to the growing need for transitional and supportive housing for people in recovery from opioid addiction and people leaving jail or prison with untreated drug problems led to the creation of the National Alliance for Recovery Residences (NARR) in 2011. NARR developed standards and a recommended certification process for state affiliates to implement and is a repository for best practices for recovery residences.[12] NARR provides four levels of certification, with the lowest level providing informal peer support and the highest level providing licensed clinical services on site. These levels of housing correspond to the needs of people at different stages of recovery. All provide an alcohol- and drug-free living environment and the social model of recovery support; many provide recovery support services (onsite meetings, structured living, links with employment, education, and volunteer opportunities); a few provide life skills development; and very few provide clinical services on site. (A full description of NARR certification requirements can be found at https://narronline.org/affiliate-services/standards-and-certification-program/.)

FINDING A RECOVERY RESIDENCE

Often, family members are looking for a recovery residence at the last moment, like when a loved one is leaving jail with no support services or is couch surfing after treatment. In moments like these, it's hard to make a good decision about housing. Doing a little homework beforehand, if possible, can help.

- It's critical to find a recovery residence that fits the needs of the person in recovery. For example, a person in early recovery, just beginning to stabilize, may need the highest level of care a recovery residence can provide, which can include clinical care. A person who has a job and is looking for peer support and accountability may need the lowest level of housing. People with a history of relapses, overdoses, mental health issues, or trauma in their lives likely will need a more structured and supportive environment.

- Most states have affiliates of the National Alliance for Recovery Residences, which certify recovery residences. If you're looking for recovery housing, the first step is to consult the state affiliate, which may have up-to-date information on certified residences. A list of NARR's state affiliates is available at www.narronline.org. A local recovery community organization also may have updated information.

- Some treatment agencies create aftercare plans that include sober living. Counselors and administrators at these agencies likely will know which houses provide quality support. They also can tap into counselors at treatment agencies in the geographic area where the person in early recovery wants to live.

- Rather than relying solely on brochures and websites, it's also a good idea to network with other families who have faced similar challenges in finding the right fit for their loved ones. It may even be possible to talk with people who have lived in the house and transitioned successfully to independent living.

If you're looking for a safe place to live in recovery, the most critical question to ask is, "Is this house certified, and if not, why not?" Here are some additional questions to ask recovery residence operators to determine if and how a house can meet your needs.

1. *Do I get a written and signed resident agreement?* This agreement should include behavior guidelines, what fees are due and when, and circumstances under which you may be asked to leave. You shouldn't waive any individual rights or fair housing rights.

2. *How do you ensure that the environment is free from alcohol and illicit drug use?* Recovery residences have different strategies, and the operator should tell you how they create a safe recovery environment.

3. *What supports are available to help me live in recovery?* The house should expect you to engage in positive relationships with other residents and people in the broader community. This could include regular house meetings, regular attendance at support groups in the community, recreational activities, and the expectation to live in the house congenially and cooperatively. Attending a support group meeting in the broader community and taking advantage of volunteer opportunities like serving food in a soup kitchen also should be encouraged if not required.

4. *Does this house feel like a home?* You should have access to a common area where residents can meet informally, and you should be able to buy, store, and prepare your own food. There should be a space for storing your personal items, and you should have access to basic utilities, hot water, and functioning appliances. Furniture should be in good shape.

5. *How do you ensure residents' safety?* The house should follow all building and fire codes; have smoke alarms, fire extinguishers, and carbon monoxide monitors; and not be overcrowded. Naloxone must be accessible, and appropriate individuals must be knowledgeable and trained in its use. Each resident should have emergency contact information readily available.

6. *What is the average length of stay in your house?* While there's no concrete evidence yet about the best length of stay, if the average is low—two months or less—this might signal that residents aren't adequately screened and need a different level of support than a

particular residence provides. It also may mean that residents are relapsing frequently and being kicked out. On the other hand, if the average is high—more than nine or ten months—this might mean that residents stay too long and don't move on in their lives to independent-living arrangements.

7. *What are the employment requirements?* Residents should be required to work, and they should be responsible for paying for their rent and food by the second or third month of living in the house. These requirements solidify their commitment to communal living and create accountability to people outside the house. (Some houses encourage residents to go to school and volunteer as well.)

8. *How many house managers are there, and how long have they been in recovery?* There should be a manager in the house at all times, and the manager should be stable in their recovery. While there is no recommended length of time, anything less than a year in recovery may not be enough to manage a residence appropriately.

9. *Is the owner of the residence involved?* Owner involvement shows an interest in the people living in the house.

10. *What is your relapse policy?* You want your loved one to be in a safe and drug-free environment, so the house should have a relapse policy that ensures that drugs will not be available. This doesn't necessarily mean that a person who relapses is automatically discharged—which might not be safe for that person—but it does mean that bringing drugs into the house and relapses are handled swiftly and with the safety of all residents in mind.

Recovery Residence Options

The range of housing options depends mostly on where you live, where the treatment facility is, the level of services you need, and how much you can afford. Most houses are gender-specific for men or women, although some co-ed houses exist. Recovery housing specifically for the trans and non-binary community is rare. Recovery residences reflect the neighborhood where they're located and the people they serve. More expensive houses are in higher-income communities for wealthier people.[13] For people with little or no means, recovery houses can be modest houses or apartments with no amenities. While spending a lot of money on an expensive recovery residence will buy a nicer house, it doesn't guarantee a smoother path to recovery or better peer support. Many humble recovery residences provide solid, lifesaving assistance.

Although recovery residences are located throughout the United States, finding a place in rural areas is nearly impossible. People in these areas often seek recovery housing elsewhere, leaving the place where they used drugs and got into trouble, in hopes of returning home later when they're stable. Some recovery housing clusters around treatment agencies, including houses owned by the facility. While this creates an effective referral mechanism and can be comforting to family members at a time of crisis—a person finishes the agency's treatment and goes directly to the agency's recovery house—it doesn't always allow for choice or create the best fit for housing. It may take time to find the right resources after treatment, and by the time everything is lined up, the person may be on the street again. It's easy to understand why family members often take whatever bed is available for their loved ones.

Most residences are well run and provide much-needed structure and support for people in early recovery; however, a few are essentially unsupervised living situations where people may use drugs or engage in other unhealthy behaviors. It's rare, but in some houses, owners extort sex from residents. Some recovery residence owners are out to make a buck, and low-quality services, overcrowding, and minimal staffing contribute to a greater likelihood for relapse and overdose. Still others deliver overly harsh penalties for breaking house rules and can do a lot of harm to vulnerable people in early recovery.

A small number of residences promote a harm reduction approach by allowing the use of cannabis, kratom, or other drugs. This harm reduction approach in housing is generally not well accepted in the recovery community.

OXFORD HOUSES:
A UNIQUE TYPE OF RECOVERY RESIDENCE

Oxford Houses are a particular type of recovery residence. The houses themselves are ordinary one-family houses that are rented, not owned, by residents. Each house is financially self-supporting and democratically run by its members. Like most other recovery residences, the Oxford House model is rooted in the 12-step recovery path. Oxford Houses accept people taking medications for addiction. Because Oxford Houses don't have a time limit for residents to be in the house, residents who would like to move from medications to abstinence have the time and support to make a successful transition.

Living in an Oxford House can create a sense of community while learning how to live independently. "Everything we did, we did together," one Oxford House resident said. "We are our own bosses, so we trust each other to make living together work. Living there, I forged friendships with women that I needed then. They really grounded me."

Recovery Housing and Medications for Addiction

As an outgrowth of AA, recovery residences were based on an abstinence-only approach to recovery; however, this is changing. The National Alliance for Recovery Residences has published guidelines for recovery residences interested in supporting people taking medications for substance use disorders, and a growing number are accepting residents on Suboxone or methadone. The guidelines include suggestions for training staff and residents about medications, developing ways to store and dispose of them, and observing residents take their medications as ways to discourage residents from diverting medications from medical use.[14, 15]

Recovery Residences and Recovery Capital

Living in a recovery residence provides a safe place to live and creates the opportunity to build recovery capital through peer support, education, and skill-building. Research shows that recovery housing contributes to recovery capital,[16] but we don't know what type of housing works best for people entering recovery. The American Society of Addiction Medicine, the leading organization for addiction medicine in the United States, has criteria for placing people in appropriate treatment programs based on their substance use disorder severity and need for services and support. To date, no such standards exist for people seeking recovery housing. Using a recovery capital scale as an initial assessment could help identify the mismatch between recovery capital and what the person needs for support. Then the person could be referred to a housing arrangement that meets those needs. Research is underway to address this issue.

Drugs in Recovery Houses

Sometimes, despite house managers' and residents' best efforts, a resident brings illicit drugs or alcohol into a recovery residence and starts using again. This tends to tarnish the reputation of all recovery residences. In most houses, managers deal with relapse by moving the individual to a higher level of support that facilitates recovery. In some poorly managed houses, though, residents who bring in drugs are kicked out with no plan for support, or no action is taken. Information about this activity isn't available publicly. It's only by word of mouth among treatment providers and the recovery community that it's possible to learn about specific residences and their ability to keep drugs out of the house. For family members looking for drug-free recovery housing for a loved one, consulting local treatment providers, asking recovery community centers that refer people to recovery housing, and networking with other families who have had a similar experience are the best ways to learn about local recovery residences' reputations.

Overdose Deaths in Recovery Houses

Sadly, sometimes people die from drug overdoses in recovery residences. It's not the norm, but it does happen. We know about overdose deaths through anecdotes, but reliable data aren't available. The recovery community is reluctant to talk about them publicly because they may reflect poorly on people in recovery in general, so we don't know the extent of deaths or the specific circumstances in which people died.

Residents of recovery houses overdose because people leaving treatment are at high risk for opioid overdose, and this is precisely the demographic of people living there. People who have used opioids—heroin, prescription painkillers, fentanyl—and then go for a while without using them have a reduced tolerance for such drugs. When they start to use again, they typically use at the same level as when they stopped, but they don't need that much to get high. The old level may be enough to shut down the central nervous system and cause death.

Another reason for opioid overdose deaths in recovery residences is that such homes didn't have naloxone on hand in the past. Sometimes referred to by its brand name, Narcan, naloxone may reverse opioid overdoses. In the past few years, laws and regulations around the use and distribution of naloxone have increased access, and many recovery residences now have it on site as a precaution. NARR certification requires that houses have naloxone on site and accessible, but because data are unavailable, we can't know if these changes have reduced overdose deaths at recovery residences.

Access to Recovery Housing

Substance use disorders affect people across all economic circumstances; however, people living in poverty face significant barriers to treatment and recovery support. Some communities have local nonprofit organizations that provide scholarships to people in need for the first month or two of rent to give them time to get on their feet and find a job. Some states provide vouchers or other types of support for recovery housing. But overall, public support for recovery housing is scant, and people without means face significant barriers. A young homeless man I interviewed to understand the needs of homeless teens seeking recovery boiled it down to the essentials: "Man, you gotta have bank to have housing."

Good Neighbors

It's in the interest of communities to support recovery housing for economic as well as humane reasons. Research shows that overall, small residences (six or fewer residents) located in residential neighborhoods add to a neighborhood's quality of life compared with doing nothing and simply ignoring drug and alcohol problems.[17]

Complaints from neighbors typically are associated with large houses or having too many houses in one area and have to do with noise, offensive language, and leaving cigarette butts outside. Because being a "good neighbor" is such an essential tenet of recovery housing, many recovery residences also distribute brochures in the neighborhood to explain what a recovery residence is, who lives there, and who to contact with questions. Individual residents may reach out to neighbors to volunteer, for example, to mow the lawn or organize a neighborhood cleanup day.

What Can Allies Do?

For Family Members and Friends

- If your loved one is in early recovery and looking for housing, ask about their housing needs and if they want you to help them find safe living options. People with a history of relapse, overdose, mental health issues, or trauma in their lives likely will need a more structured and supportive environment. Do your homework to find NARR-certified houses, even if they're not as close to home as you'd like.

- Finding housing isn't the same as finding a home. You can help by understanding what "home" means to your loved ones, and, if they want some assistance, helping to create that wherever they are living by assisting with clothing, bedding, groceries, or books, depending on house rules.

- Abide by rules of recovery residences to support new structure and accountability in their lives, such as "no cell phones" and "no boyfriends." You can model your new relationship with your loved one in recovery by setting boundaries consistent with the residence's requirements.

For Everyone

- Learn why recovery housing is essential, and find out what is available in your town or city and what's happening in your state regarding access to safe housing.

- If recovery housing exists in your town, help combat the stigma against recovery housing by promoting the positive effects of having a recovery house in the neighborhood.

- Join local housing coalitions that address homelessness and affordable housing coalitions and groups that focus on creating resources for people released from jail or prison, and advocate for recovery housing.

For Community Organizations

- If you want to start a recovery residence in your community, don't assume you know how to do it. Consult people with experience such as house operators and managers to create the right mix of structure, accountability, volunteer opportunities, and other vital aspects of the social model of recovery.

- Be sure to include conversations about the need for recovery residences in existing coalitions that address homelessness, affordable housing, and reentry resources for people released from jail or prison. Invite people in recovery to join these coalitions.

- Reach out and create partnerships with recovery houses to link residents with legal aid, credit, and financial management services. Banks may be interested in this activity, in part as a local service and in part because many recovery house residents have debt that banks and credit unions can help restructure.

- Offer volunteer opportunities to recovery house residents as ways for them to give back, integrate into the community, and develop new and healthy interests and relationships.

- Create scholarships that benefit people living in recovery residences.

For Employers

- Reach out to recovery residences with employment and job training opportunities.

- Host a recovery job fair and invite everyone living in recovery residences.

For Municipal Leaders

- Understand the status of recovery residences under federal and state laws so you can explain to citizens the rights of recovery residents and the restrictions on recovery housing. Understand the interplay of local ordinances and state and federal laws to avoid violating the Fair Housing Act or the Americans with Disabilities Act.

- Be part of the national conversation on policies that support safe recovery housing.

For Landlords and Property Management Companies

- If you're interested in launching a recovery house or houses, don't assume that recovery housing is like any other housing project. Start by contacting NARR or your state's affiliate for helpful information. Consult people with experience as house operators and managers to create the right mix of structure, accountability, volunteer opportunities, and other vital aspects of the social model of recovery.

- If you rent to recovery residents, help reduce stigma by sharing your experiences and becoming a spokesperson for people in recovery, including at local landlord associations.

16

CHALLENGES TO
FINDING SAFE HOUSING

IN 2014, I conducted a focus group with eight men and three women in early recovery. The local treatment program was interested in learning more about what recovery support services would be most helpful. Focus group participants were in early recovery, and they were very clear about what helped them, and safe housing was included in that list. (The others were having a supportive family member, a community of peers, and professional counselors.)

After getting out of the county jail, John lived in supportive housing, a combination of housing and support services for people who experience homelessness or mental illness, that offered ongoing counseling, job training, life skills education, and other services for six months after leaving the jail. He credits his probation officer with helping him turn his life around. "After I got out, he gave me more chances than I can count," John says. "He didn't lock me up again—he helped me." John tears up when he talks about his mother, who travels more than one hundred miles every week to bring his daughter to visit. "My daughter is back in my life. I never thought I would be allowed to see her again." John says that for people used to making decisions based on "getting drugs and fighting every day just to find something to eat," finding a new place to live and creating a healthy lifestyle are almost impossible without help.

Dick, a clean-shaven fifty-year-old, lived in an apartment with five other men in recovery. He described this sober living arrangement as a "bridge between rehab and your life, a place to live with a support system, where people understand what you're going through, to help you get back on your feet." He'd been sober and living with his family for more than a decade when he started drinking again. Within months, his wife kicked him out of the house. He knew enough from his past experiences that he needed help, and he checked himself into a residential treatment program. After a month there, he moved to the apartment. "When you leave rehab," he said, "you need a little more, something extra to help you through."

Monica started her recovery in jail. She received support from women in a Therapeutic Community program run by the jail. "They taught me a lot and gave me hope. I didn't know I was a person with a problem when I was using actively. I didn't understand the nature of addiction, didn't know there was help for my hopeless situation." Now she lives in a recovery residence for women in a small town, and she is outspoken about the needs of women in recovery. "Women need women as part of their support system," she says. "There's a huge gap when it comes to services and support—going from the safe environment in treatment back to the community without support is a huge gap. People fresh out of jail or rehab don't know what to do or where to go. There's just not much for women."

All of this is consistent with current literature on recovery, showing that people in residential treatment are more successful if they have recovery support services, including access to safe housing, when they complete treatment or leave jail or prison.[1] Informal sober living arrangements like Dick's in the apartment and more structured recovery residences like Monica's are the most common housing options. Supportive housing like John lived in is for people with needs for support beyond what peers can offer. Historically, this housing was usually for people who experienced homelessness and mental illness, but it is increasingly available for people with addiction. Supportive housing is in short supply in most cities and towns.

Finding Housing with a Criminal Record

Kayla's experience looking for suitable housing after leaving jail is all too common. "I love my life, and I love recovery," Kayla said when I asked her about her living situation, "but there are struggles." She spent fifteen months in a shabby duplex after leaving jail. "Now I'm in public housing, which is a nice place to live. But people are using [drugs] there, too."

Kayla's mother Tammy provided some background: When Kayla was in high school, Tammy managed tense situations at home by finding relatives who'd take

Kayla in when the family just couldn't deal with the conflicts and chaos created by Kayla's drug use. Tammy didn't want to go into detail, but she made sure I knew that Kayla was never homeless. She lived with her grandparents off and on for years, where there was always a place to sleep.

About a month before Kayla's scheduled release from jail, her case manager gave her information on housing options. Together, they filled out paperwork for federal support for housing and openings at a local public housing agency. Kayla was nervous about what would happen when she was released. She and her boyfriend were planning to live together, but they didn't have an apartment lined up. They both had criminal records, and she was afraid that they wouldn't find a place. Kayla also was scared that she would start using again if she left jail without a safe place to live. She'd seen that happen to friends, and she knew she didn't want to return to that life. One of her close friends had died from a drug overdose shortly after leaving prison.

When Kayla went to the public housing agency to find out about her housing voucher, she learned that the case manager hadn't sent in the paperwork. Kayla was stunned and discouraged. "It wasn't the case manager's fault," Kayla said. "She was busy and had too many women to help." But it was just one more setback and one more item on a growing to-do list of creating her life in recovery. Kayla filed the paperwork, expecting to wait for weeks or months for approval, and looked for housing she could afford without outside financial help.

"Looking for an apartment was hard," Kayla said. She and her boyfriend had enough money for the security deposit and the first month's rent, but they both had criminal records. Time and again, landlords turned them down for "nice apartments" after a background check turned up their criminal convictions. Living with relatives wasn't an option, so Kayla worked through her parents' networks in town to find a studio in a filthy, low-cost motel that rented by the week. People were actively using drugs in the dingy studios nearby. "We were there for two weeks, and when we found a place that would take us without a background check, we signed the lease on the spot," Kayla explained.

The duplex they found was substandard: leaks in the ceiling ruined their furniture, mold accumulated on the walls and their clothing, and the little bugs that fed on the mold invaded all the rooms. Kayla and her boyfriend lived there for fifteen months, constantly battling with the landlord to fix the leaks. While they were there, they had a baby who spent her first three months living in that moldy, bug-infested space.

"You don't want to do it, but you have to," Kayla explained. She wanted the best for her daughter, but all she could manage was a substandard duplex. She wanted something better for herself, too, but she had to accept the situation and continue to look for better options.

On the day we spoke, she was moving into public housing. Her application had finally been accepted. For Kayla, every day since being released has been a balancing act to stay sober, stay in school, repair relationships with her family, and be a good partner and mother. Her struggles with the landlord, living with leaks and broken fixtures, and staying warm in the winter in a drafty duplex, added stress. She could have reverted to old habits of using drugs to cope. Instead, she pushed ahead, met the challenges, and accepted the setbacks.

"I started looking for a safe and affordable place to live the day I was released. Fifteen months later, I finally have a place."

People coming out of jail or prison may have a difficult time finding a place to live. Most prisons and jails have meager resources to link people being released to any type of housing, let alone housing that supports a new life in recovery. So, people leaving incarceration may not know about available options. If they're in a relationship, like Kayla, they may not be eligible for a recovery residence. Many women's houses prohibit partner relationships, and recovery housing for couples is sparse. If they look for housing in the rental market, having a history of convictions creates an enormous barrier to renting housing that meets minimal standards for physical safety.

The Fair Housing Act created seven categories of protected individuals. It prohibits discrimination in the sale, rental, or financing of housing based on color (of skin), disability, familial status, national origin, race, religion, and sex.[2] People in recovery from substance use disorder are included in the class of people with disabilities and are protected from discrimination. However, as Kayla learned, at that time, a landlord could use discretion and refuse to rent to a person with a history of convictions. This changed in 2016 when the federal Department of Housing and Urban Development issued guidelines for rental housing (public or private). The guidelines advise landlords that they violate the Fair Housing Act if they use past convictions to restrict a person from renting without considering the severity of the crime or the time that has elapsed since it occurred. Restricting rentals based on, for example, violent crimes or crimes involving weapons or sex are permitted so long as these restrictions are applied consistently. The guidelines address the disparate impact that rental restrictions based on conviction history have had on "people of a particular race, national origin, or other protected class." In other words, the guidelines address, in part, the impact that the disproportionate arrests, convictions, and incarceration of people of color have on their opportunities for safe housing.[3]

SUBSIDIZED HOUSING OPTIONS

Families like Kayla's often find themselves working through their personal networks and looking online for affordable housing. Public housing, private low-income housing, and federal housing vouchers are other options for income-eligible people. Every community is different, so it pays to explore all options in your community.

The US Department of Housing and Urban Development's Housing Choice Vouchers Program (sometimes called "Section 8") is the federal government's housing assistance program for low-income families, the elderly, and the disabled. It helps people in those groups afford safe housing in the private market. People are responsible for finding their housing, then landlords receive the rent subsidy. This option is available only for housing in which the owner agrees to participate in the program.

Public housing authorities also provide housing opportunities for low- to moderate-income households. Rent is usually capped at 30 percent of total income. Waiting lists are often long for public housing. Information on these programs is available at your local public housing agency. For a list of agencies by state, go to www.hud.gov/program_offices/public _indian_housing/pha/contacts.

Private low-income housing is available in many communities. Some landlords offer properties at rents proportional to the tenant's income in exchange for tax credits.

Safe Housing for Women with Children

Carolyn is a cheerful woman in her fifties who knows what it's like to seek treatment and recovery with young children. Now she's a successful businesswoman and active in Maine's recovery movement. Her alcohol use disorder and drug addiction created chaos in her life, and she wasn't able to take care of herself or her children. Her path to recovery included an intervention with the state Department of Health and Human Services, and she went to inpatient treatment while her mother and sister took care of her children. Carolyn eventually moved to McAuley Residence, a program for women with children. A group of Catholic nuns started McAuley in the 1980s, and it's now a collaboration of a hospital system, public housing, and the Catholic Church. At the time, the house had three small apartments, but today it has moved to a new location and has grown to serve twenty-five women with children, a testament to the increased need for structured living for women in recovery and their children.

"I didn't know anything," Carolyn explained. "I needed guidance. With kids, it wasn't just me I had to worry about. I knew what not to do, but I didn't know what to do." At McAuley, Carolyn received the guidance and structure she needed to live independently with her children. Gradually, she built up her parenting skills, and after nine months, they came to live with her in her two-bedroom apartment at McAuley.

"It was a beautiful, safe place," Carolyn remembered. Two women on staff worked with her on life skills—cooking, managing, and parenting skills. She is especially grateful to them. "They took care of me." Carolyn tears up as she remembers. "They helped me understand that I could be a good parent."

Carolyn worked in publishing and was a whiz at computers before she was in treatment, and she was able to work professionally while she was at McAuley. The support she received included childcare. Without childcare, she says, she wouldn't have been able to put her life back together. "Childcare is a big part of my recovery. I can't say that loud enough," Carolyn says. "That's support that is lacking today." Without childcare, it's hard to go to school or work or go to support groups, and young women struggle to maintain custody of their children and rebuild their lives.

Three years after she first entered rehab, Carolyn had her children back full-time. McAuley Residence held the rent she paid in an account for her to use when she left. After living there for twelve months, she bought a house and moved in with her children, and she still lives there two decades later.

SUPPORTIVE HOUSING

Homelessness and recovery rarely go hand in hand. Drugs and alcohol are readily available on the street and often in homeless shelters. Housing models that address homelessness or housing instability and substance use disorder (and mental health) include the "housing first model," which doesn't require abstinence to obtain housing and other support, and "permanent supportive housing," which may or may not require abstinence to be housed and receive other services. These housing models provide a higher level of support and services, including addiction treatment and case management, than recovery residences.[4]

What Can Allies Do?

Finding safe housing is especially challenging for parents with children, people with mental health issues, and people leaving jail or prison. As caring community members, we can help people in recovery integrate or reintegrate into our community by making sure we have safe housing options. In addition to supporting recovery residences in our neighborhoods, we can work with landlords to decrease stigma and discrimination against people with past convictions and improve the quality of rental units. Community coalitions that can ensure fair access to affordable housing and community agencies can work together to establish supportive housing projects.

For Family Members

- Everyone has networks in the community. If your loved one wants you to, use yours to find safe housing for them.

- If you have a family member in early recovery who has children, especially young children, ask if they would like you to babysit. Critical times for babysitting include when your loved one is looking for housing or a job, needs to go to counseling or medical appointments, or just needs a break from childcare.

- If your loved one is looking for independent living, ask if they would like you to help them sort out options for public benefits, like housing vouchers. Go with them to see apartments, and use your voice to support them when landlords or property management company representatives question their conviction background. If substandard housing is their only option, help them improve their living situation whenever possible by offering to repair broken fixtures and contact the landlord for help with other issues.

For Community Organizations

- Social services agencies and faith-based groups can set up supportive housing and wraparound services, especially for women with children. This can require enormous effort on the part of local community organizations, authorities and agencies, and public and private funders and needs lots of planning and coordination to develop long-term solutions.

- Make sure housing for people in recovery who have a history of convictions or are raising children is part of discussions about homelessness and supportive housing. Invite people in recovery to join housing coalitions, listen to their stories, and pay attention to their suggestions for programs that will help people who are struggling.

For Landlords

- Get informed! Learn about your own biases in renting to people with a conviction record, and figure out how you can contribute to a positive conversation about renting to people in recovery.

- The interplay of the Fair Housing Act, local zoning ordinances, and state housing requirements can be complex and confusing. Reach out to your statewide landlords' association to learn more.

SECTION 6
The Pillars of Recovery: Purpose

17

EMPLOYMENT

MIKE'S FAMILY TRIED to help him with his substance use disorder many times, but early attempts didn't lead to recovery. "I wasn't in a good recovery situation," Mike said. "I'd clean up and get a job, and then I'd start using all over again. It just didn't work." He had been in and out of residential treatment in New York since he was seventeen, and by the time he was twenty-three, he found himself homeless on the boardwalk in Norfolk, Virginia. His brother was stationed there in the Navy, and he helped Mike get connected with the McShin Foundation, the recovery community organization in nearby Richmond, a city known for its recovery support services. "That's where I finally found a good recovery situation," Mike said. "I got connected to John Shinholser at McShin, and he let me stay in one of their recovery residences for a night. The next day, he found a bed in a treatment center and drove me there. When I was done, he picked me up, drove me to Richmond, and offered me a place in another recovery residence. He helped me every step of the way when I couldn't help myself. He saved my life."

Staff at McShin found part-time work for him doing manual labor. He became good friends with John Lowndes, owner of Hurricane Fence, which installs fencing and perimeter security solutions, through the recovery community. In 2010, Lowndes offered him a full-time job several months later. "He hired a lot of people in recovery," Mike said. "What I learned working there was that, when we're in recovery, we tend to work pretty damned hard. We feel an obligation to put a good effort forth. So, I learned how to work and how to connect with the people I was working with. I saw effort, teamwork, and unity when I worked there. It was so much fun and so beneficial to have camaraderie, a bond, and to be around other people."

About a third of the employees were in recovery at that time, and everyone else in the company knew their stories. "They accepted us," Mike says. "That helped change stigma at the worksite. They learned from us that there's a part of addiction when you choose to use, but nobody chooses to be a heroin addict. They end up there, and that's where the disease comes in. When people learn that part of it, they start to understand, and that helps stigma. Now they see that people in recovery operate like other people. They see me. They see me with my kids and my wife, who is also in recovery.

"I'm open with my situation," Mike continues. "I don't need to hide a whole lot. You never know when someone needs help. So many times, someone comes to me privately and says, 'Hey, can you help me with my friend or my dad or my child?'

"It's amazing and scary how much people hide their problems," Mike says, talking about stigma. "I found out that I had a cousin in recovery for twenty years, and no one in my family told me. No one connected me to him when I was just start-ing my recovery. That could have been so helpful. Now, though, that's changed. We talk about addiction in my family."

Now Mike co-owns Hurricane Fence, which has grown to employ more than sev-enty people. Mike is enthusiastic about hiring people in recovery. "As an employer, I think the best thing I can do is push the envelope and continue to bring in people in recovery, give them an opportunity."

Mike understands what researchers have found: that employment is an essential aspect of recovery for many people. "Employment is a proven route to recovery," he says. "It's not a quick fix, and it's hard, but it can work. The hardest thing for me was to get out of my own way. I didn't do anything special. I stayed with the people in recovery. Of course, I wanted to quit my job. Of course, I wanted to get paid more. But I could talk to other people in recovery, and they'd say, 'Let's see how your spirit settles, and then you can decide what you want to do.'"

Why do we work? Many of us say we work because we need money for housing, food, school, transportation, and generally getting by every day. But usually, we have other motivations as well. Most of us work to find an iden-tity, meaning, and purpose, be part of a team, have opportunities for learning and growth, and contribute to society.[1] We find satisfaction in working with others, learning new skills, accomplishing a task, learning about ourselves and our definition of success, setting goals, and reaching them. Work can be a source of dignity. In all these domains, employment builds recovery capi-tal. Some people in recovery feel an added motivation to be employed and valuable because, for the years of their active addiction, they felt as if they were "takers" from society and want a chance to be "givers."

Employers have every incentive to create supportive environments for people in recovery. The costs of substance use in the workplace include higher health care costs, missed work, unscheduled leave, and higher turnover. Research shows that health care costs are lower for people in recovery than people with untreated substance use disorder (SUD). The same holds true for their family members. In terms of worker turnover, people in recovery stay with one employer at about the same rates as other workers. They take less unscheduled leave than their peers with untreated SUDs. In fact, they take even fewer days of unscheduled leave than workers in their industry who have never had a SUD. The costs of a SUD vary by industry. For example, the extra cost to employers in the construction industry for each worker with untreated SUD is $2,689. In the information and communications industry, the extra cost per worker is $13,534. The average for all industries is $6,643.[2]

Research

Research shows that employment contributes significantly to recovery capital by providing access to independent housing and health insurance, easing financial worries, and improving social standing. Employment also may provide needed daily structure, increase self-esteem and happiness, and enhance quality of life. Having a job can play an important role in relapse prevention, too.[3] Studies show that employment is as good a predictor of maintained recovery as treatment duration—longer stays in treatment point to good treatment outcomes, and so does having employment after treatment.[4]

WORK AND VOLUNTEER OPPORTUNITIES FOR RESTORATIVE ACTION

Sometimes, volunteer opportunities can be as effective as paid work in building recovery capital and creating opportunities for participating in community life in early recovery. For example, Sarah Coupe, a woman in long-term recovery, runs three women's recovery residences in Portland,

Maine. One of them, Grace House, is an old, single-family home in a quiet neighborhood in the city. Sarah lives downstairs with her husband, two children, and their dog. On the second and third floors, six bedrooms house twelve women in early recovery. The kitchen has cubbies for each woman's food, bulletin boards with the week's schedule, words of inspiration and encouragement, and a dog-walking schedule. A meditation room near the kitchen with two chairs and a colorful mandala painted on the wall is where women can be quiet, explore their thoughts, and learn about their new lives. A big yard is a place for women to play with their children, have cookouts, and sit in evening meetings around the firepit.

"Women in Grace House are from all over New England. They come with the consequences of their addiction—lost work, broken families, debt, court fines, and jail time," Sarah says. "They come to this house to be healed. People need so much more now, more than just a weekly meeting with their sponsor. That's the old AA. They need the community of the house to heal from the soul-sickness of society. One of the ways they heal is by 'giving back,' by volunteering. That's why the weekly schedule includes volunteering at a local nonprofit that distributes donated clothing to people in need, which is an integral part of their recovery journey. They learn to think of others and understand how they are part of something bigger than themselves. Expecting someone whose life has become unmanageable to turn it around on their own—that very rarely happens. Volunteering like this is a chance to merge broken souls with healing opportunities."

Barriers to Employment

Employment is a critical building block in recovery, especially in the early months, including during treatment. Even though we know that employment boosts recovery capital, finding work can be a tremendous challenge. People in recovery often have a poor employment history, limited educational experience, or a history of convictions that shut the door to many job opportunities. Current parole and probation requirements can limit availability to work. Mental and physical problems can make it hard to maintain

a required work schedule. Limited education, job skills, and work experience reduce the types of work people are eligible for. People in recovery
also may lack "soft skills" like a work ethic that includes showing up to work
on time every day, professionalism in work settings, problem-solving skills,
and good communication.[5]

The local economic climate and social environment also create limitations.
Substance use disorders hit low-income people the hardest. Living in areas
where unemployment is high means few job opportunities regardless of individual capabilities and experience. Even though employers may not discriminate based on disability—being in recovery from substance use disorder is a
disability under the Americans with Disabilities Act—stigma and discrimination in the real-life hiring process and at the worksite mean many people
in recovery never get a chance to try their hand at work.[6] In addition to social
stigma, employers may shy away from people with a history of a substance use
disorder, fearing higher medical and workers' compensation costs, higher job
turnover, and fewer days worked.[7]

BAN THE BOX

"Have you ever been arrested or convicted of a crime? Check yes or
no." Chances are, if you've filled out a standard job application form,
you've had to answer that question. Employers use the answer to weed
out applicants with a history of arrests and convictions. Those applications typically go immediately to the "no" pile regardless of whether the
arrest led to a conviction, the circumstances when the crime occurred,
or what the applicant has done since then. Online services that provide
employers with quick background checks have made this process easy,
but the data underlying the database these services use aren't complete
and usually aren't reliable.

Having a record of convictions is a significant barrier to employment
for many people in recovery. Some states, counties, and cities have passed
"ban-the-box" laws and policies prohibiting employers from asking questions about arrest and conviction history in the initial application. Some
federal legislators have contemplated enacting federal laws to encourage

all states to do the same. Such laws have the potential to help a massive swath of the American workforce—including people in recovery—since 77.7 million, or one in three, working-age adults in the United States has been arrested.[8]

Employment-Based Recovery Services

From an employer's perspective, alcohol and drug problems are a hefty cost of doing business. The annual economic impact of substance use in the United States is more than \$578 billion (not counting tobacco use). Lost productivity—employees not working to their full potential when they're on the job or not showing up at all—makes up a large portion of that.[9] Around 70 percent of people who use drugs, binge drinkers, and heavy drinkers are employed full- or part-time, so employers have a big stake in creating a work environment that encourages and supports employees looking for help on the road to recovery.[10]

Employment-based recovery services come in many forms. People in early recovery with many unmet needs may be in a treatment program that provides case management that coordinates clinical services, recovery housing, childcare, and employment. Less intensive treatment programs may provide job-search assistance, help writing resumes, and assistance preparing for job interviews. Local recovery community organizations often offer these same forms of assistance.

Employers don't have to have a special program to support employees in recovery and their families. One small employer in Maine, recognized for being a solid ally of people in recovery, put it this way: "I didn't set out to be recovery friendly. I just wanted to do the right thing for my employees. It turned out that many of them are in early recovery." As a small employer, he made sure they got the training they needed, flexible work hours, peer support, health insurance, and a safe space to talk about their recovery. He celebrated their recovery milestones with their friends and family and encouraged them in difficult times.

Some large employers offer programs to help their employees and family members access treatment and support, often through Employee Assistance Programs and health insurance plans. Most employers recognize that they don't know everything about recovery. They can't provide the support that peers can, so they partner with recovery community organizations to link employees to peer services, sponsor or fund training programs for people in recovery to gain job skills, and hold job fairs. Some businesses, often established by people in recovery, place employing people in recovery at the heart of their business model.

Recovery Friendly Workplaces

Motivated by the economic and human costs of untreated addiction, some twenty state governments have created Recovery Friendly Workplace programs. These reflect a shift in thinking from taking disciplinary action when an employee has a problem with drugs or alcohol to creating an environment that focuses on help, hope, and the potential of healthy employees. Recovery Friendly Workplace programs assign a designation for employers that meet specific requirements, like committing to a stigma-free workplace; connecting with local recovery support services; providing information about substance use, mental health, and wellness to employees; and providing education and training to supervisors, so they know how to support people in recovery.[11] In addition, recovery-friendly employers make sure their health insurance benefits include sufficient substance use and mental health counseling, residential treatment, and medication-assisted treatment. Beyond these general commitments, Recovery Friendly Workplaces typically focus on retaining employees and building skills specific to individual employee needs. The goal of Recovery Friendly Workplaces is to create healthy and safe environments where people in recovery can thrive.

RECOVERY JOB FAIRS

Employers and employer organizations like chambers of commerce and Rotary Clubs can support recovery by hosting recovery job fairs, where local employers looking for employees connect with people in recovery looking for work. Recovery community centers can be essential partners, promoting the fair and arranging transportation. Employers can make presentations and hold trainings to introduce fairgoers to the types of work available and on-the-job training opportunities. Local community colleges and vocational schools can also participate by holding resume workshops and creating a connection between courses offered and possible jobs. Recovery job fairs also create an opportunity for the recovery community center staff and others to make presentations and educate employers about recovery.

Recovery-Friendly Employers

Kennebunk Savings (KS) is a designated Recovery Friendly Workplace in New Hampshire. Liz Torrance, community relations and social responsibility manager, described the bank's motivation behind seeking the designation. "Our employees are our most important resource; they are vital to our success, and this is one of the ways we can support them," she says. "In addition to supporting our own employees, we also wanted to be a resource to other employers, to take a leadership role in the business community and stress that supporting people in recovery is everyone's job." Leadership started with the president of the bank and its board of directors. The president and CEO, Bradford C. Paige, began by talking with the board of directors. They supported the work immediately. One of the directors had a family member in active addiction. He spoke openly about the problem with his family member, who was the same age as the other directors' children. It was the first time he had discussed this at a board meeting. He created a unifying moment when he said, "I'm 100 percent behind anything we do with substance use disorder."

The first step was for KS staff assigned to the program to learn how to connect with local resources like treatment programs, recovery residences, and support groups. Next, they reached out to local recovery community centers. Finally, they created a resource list that they distributed in open and visible places and in less visible areas for people who wanted to be discreet.

Then they worked on changing workplace culture. They started by training managers and creating "frequently asked questions," preparing them to
respond appropriately when they learned of an employee's substance use
problem or the struggles a family was having with a loved one in addiction.
"You deal with people with substance use disorder the same way you deal
with any other health issue, like diabetes, if someone comes to you with a concern," Liz said. "So much of what we did is about addressing stigma, teaching
our workforce that substance use disorder is a health problem, recovery is a
strength—not a weakness, and we want to help people get better."

At one point in the process, working with their colleagues at other institutions in the community, they realized that "not everyone is interested in doing
this work. Some people have no appetite for it," Brad said. "I'd never even
thought of working on this as being a stigma for the bank until we brought in
a marketing group for a public forum, and one of the marketing people con-
gratulated us for taking a 'big risk' by putting ourselves out there. Honestly,
it never occurred to me. I thought it was a problem to be solved, and we were
going to do what we could to help address it.

"Next, we wanted to make sure we had the healthiest environment for
employees, so we reviewed our policies. We made sure our Employee Assistance Program could support people who might seek help for themselves or
family members. We worked with our human resources team to consider federal laws such as the Americans with Disabilities Act. Finally, we checked our
health insurance benefits to be sure employees have access to mental health
counseling and treatment. We didn't need to make any changes, but it was an
excellent opportunity to work together and talk about substance use disorder
and recovery.

"We also created an opportunity for everybody at all levels of the bank to
take action. This was important. We wanted to be sure everyone knew they
had a part to play. One thing we did early on was to give out bags for safe prescription drug disposal to our customers, for free, in all of our bank lobbies
and at our internal operations center. This got customers and bank tellers
engaged in a very hands-on way. And it's a practice we continue today."

When the team had laid this groundwork for their Recovery Friendly Workplace program, Brad launched the program through an email to all employees.
He immediately received emails from employees who had experiences with

substance use disorder, a person whose mother had died from an overdose, employees whose children are in recovery, and people who want to help. Now KS is working on next steps, fully committed to continuing its journey as long as its resources can continue to make a difference.

Hiring People in Early Recovery

"Recovery is recovery," Margo Walsh tells me. "But you can't lump all substances into one bucket. People coming out of heroin or opioid addiction live in a different world than people with alcohol use disorder." Margo founded and runs MaineWorks, a construction and landscaping staffing company with a social mission. The company, a B Corp, provides dignified employment for people recovering from substance use disorder and people with felony convictions. After they've worked there for a while, stabilized in their recovery, and gained some work skills, then they can work on what they want to do in the future, on their hopes and dreams. Margo explains her company this way: "MaineWorks is the necessary middleman for the guy who is suffering and the company who needs help.

"With heroin addiction, there's typically a criminal element," Margo explains. At least 70 percent of her employees have either been arrested, gone to jail, or had their charges reduced or dropped because their parents had the means to hire an attorney. Most started using drugs at an early age.

"They were the kids who had behavioral issues and defiant behavior. They were 'other than normal,' the outsiders," Margo says. "They found pot or drinking that gave them a place to belong, and then, well, at twenty-three, they're either dead or in recovery. So, you have a twentysomething who has never been successful and can no longer medicate. They start with nothing. For the people MaineWorks hires, it's not about 'rehabilitation,' but about 'abilitation.'

"It's imperative that companies understand that people with severe opioid use disorder need so much more than other people in recovery. The job only provides financial viability. They need so much more. Over the years, they've created a lifestyle out of the hustle, and you have to unteach that. You have to hold their feet to the fire because they haven't been successful at work before. People coming from the morass of opioid use disorder need an intentional partnership with their employer. They're at high risk for relapse, and they're in constant need of support."

About half of the people who start at MaineWorks are gone after two weeks. "They showed up, put their best foot forward, and despite their best intentions, they can't stay for two weeks." But, Margo says, "for those who do stay, nearly two-thirds convert to living successfully in stable housing with stable employment. Despite incredible odds, a lot of these people who are new to the workforce get up at five o'clock, get ready, get outside even in the Maine winter, and we drive them to the job site. We help lower the barriers for people getting to work. We're part of a growing social enterprise ecosystem where we use business to solve social problems. The government and non-profits can't solve everything.

"Running this kind of business isn't for everybody," Margo says. She's in recovery herself, and she understands where her employees are coming from. "Creating a supportive environment for people who've been in recovery for years, or who didn't have the life consequences of opioid addiction, that's one thing. But you have to open your doors wider if you're really going to employ the full spectrum of people in recovery."

What Can Allies Do?

Employment is an essential building block of recovery. Understanding the specific barriers in your community can help you understand intervention points where communities can act to make it easier for people in recovery to get a job, keep the job, and advance and learn on the job.

For Everyone

- If you know someone who has started a new job or gone back to an old job after treatment, offer words of encouragement about the importance of work and the path to wellness that it supports. Talk about their recovery capital, and congratulate them on adding to it by working.

- If you know someone in recovery who is working and struggling, ask if they're open to talking about it. Perhaps they have too many stressors and need help with time management, childcare, or fixing their car. If they're open to help, do what you can or offer to find someone who can.

For Employers

- Reach out to the recovery community, for example by contacting a local recovery community center, to learn more about recovery generally and about specific employment barriers people in recovery face in your community.

- Consider your hiring process. If you automatically discard applications from people with a history of arrests and convictions or scanty work history, consider a different approach. Develop interview questions that help you understand the circumstances of the arrest and conviction and when it occurred. In addition to asking what job skills a person has, ask what they would like to learn.

- If you notice that some employees lack "soft skills" like communication, showing up on time, and professionalism, ask if they'd like a mentor and find someone willing to walk beside them as they learn these new skills.

- Consider your own workplace culture and whether people in recovery feel safe and supported. If not, consider some of the steps that lead to a Recovery Friendly Workplace, like learning about substance use disorder and teaching your employees about the importance of acceptance and hope for people who are struggling. Your local recovery community center can give you a list of resources in your area, which you can pass on to your employees. Include support groups for family members on the list.

- Look at recovery activities in your community and find ways to participate. For example, attend community meetings or sponsor recovery rallies and let your employees know you want to be a visible recovery ally. Offer to host a recovery job fair.

- Ask your employees what would help them the most. If you've established a safe environment to talk about health issues, including substance use, try one-on-one conversations to see if there's anything you can do to help.

- Find your niche. If you're a small employer, you may not have resources like Employee Assistance Programs for your employees.

Still, you may have a tight-knit group of people who know how to support each other if they understand how many people in their community are impacted by substance use disorder. If you're a large employer, you may be able to leverage resources to be designated a recovery-friendly employer.

- Check out recovery-friendly initiatives. Connecticut and New Hampshire share their resources freely. Consider turning to industry associations, insurance companies, and local chambers of commerce for resources.

- If you're considering a business venture based solely on hiring people in early recovery, make sure you know what you're doing. Having good intentions without extensive experience in this field may lead to a failed business and employees without enough support to succeed.

18

EDUCATION

ANDREW GREW UP in a wealthy family that valued education, but he wasn't interested. "Sure, my mom stressed the importance of education," he says, "but I wasn't listening." Living in an affluent community was, in fact, a source for his self-loathing and self-medication. "I grew to hate the wealth and the casual attitude toward life in my community. I hated the hypocrisy. People in wealthy communities have problems, but where I lived, they hid them. It all felt shallow and meaningless, and I didn't want to be a part of it." So, Andrew used drugs and alcohol to set himself apart, calm the pain and depression from traumatic events in early childhood, and bury his self-hatred.

Andrew finished high school and started college, but a back injury from a fall on the ice changed the course of his life. His doctor prescribed painkillers, which immediately took away the external physical pain and silenced the internal emotional racket. "I fell head over heels when given opioids. Once a collegiate athlete, I become a prisoner in my home and mind, unable to leave either without them."[1] When the doctor abruptly stopped prescribing the painkillers, Andrew turned to heroin rather than face the physical agony of opioid withdrawal and a return to a chaotic inner life. His heroin use continued for a few years, with intermittent trips to detox and residential treatment. His family stuck by him, trying time and again to help. The last time, his sister drove him from Massachusetts to a treatment facility in New Hampshire. "Something changed there," he says. "The accumulation of all of those attempts at sobriety ended with me quitting for good and entering long-term recovery."

Andrew moved to a recovery residence in Portland, Maine, and started taking a course at the University of Southern Maine (USM) when he was three months sober. "I got advice to take something I was interested in, so I took a history course. The next semester I took three courses. Then I enrolled as a full-time student. Starting slow was a good idea. It would have been hard to be a full-time student in early recovery while I was working on mental and physical health issues." Those first months in school weren't easy. "I was terrified to walk across campus. I didn't know how to be a college student without drugs or alcohol. I had some college credits, and I knew what to expect in terms of workload, but socially I was lost." However, the men in the recovery residence gave him support and encouragement, and he met some other students in recovery who helped him navigate college life in sobriety.

For Andrew, going back to college wasn't just about accruing credits for graduation. It meant a philosophical shift in his thinking. "For people in active substance use disorder and people who are starting recovery, the lens they are looking through is short term. Being able to keep attention in short bursts, being able to understand the long-term impact and long-term investment of college was a really profound thing for me." His first year as a full-time student coincided with an explosion of recovery advocacy in Portland. He got involved in forming the first chapter of Young People in Recovery in Maine and the ROCC (Recovery Oriented Campus Center) at USM.

"My recovery was and is about trying new stuff, doing new stuff, being out there as a recovery advocate," Andrew explains. So, he wouldn't say no when I suggested starting a Collegiate Recovery Program in 2016 at USM. "I was on board even though I was super busy with schoolwork and recovery advocacy. I blame you, Alison," he says with a laugh. "I blame you! I wanted to do it, and it needed to happen, and it was already happening, but I was terrified of the amount of work it was going to take. You said, 'Don't worry about it, let's do it,' and you were right. Everybody went the extra distance to make it happen."

A group of students in recovery had already been meeting informally on campus for several months, and that group took on the project. Substance use counselors employed by USM at the university health and counseling center and the dean of students joined forces. Together, they submitted a proposal to the president to create Maine's first Collegiate Recovery Program. "It felt good to see people not only appreciate the work we put in but to understand the profound and long-term impact of what we were doing," Andrew says.

Andrew explains what it was like in those first few years of college. "While I was in school and doing all the advocacy work at the same time, family and friends would frequently express concern that I was doing too much, and often they were right. But it all got done. I was doing things to stay healthy, and I started looking at the opportunities as professional development and playing the long game. The philosophical shift that happened around the same time that all of those opportunities were happening was really important for me," Andrew says. "I had a new perspective around work and opportunities. Schoolwork wasn't just homework that had to be done. It was part of the long-term benefits of college that could impact future employment. So, I could see how my recovery was going to impact my education and employment. Getting a handle on the long-term investment was a really challenging but super important piece of the puzzle."

Andrew made his mark at USM. The university president acknowledged this when Andrew graduated with a degree in chemistry. "He shakes my hand, presents a degree, and gives me a huge hug, and says, 'We're so incredibly proud of you, Andrew, and you should be so, so proud. Thank you for everything you've done here at USM, and congratulations! You did it!'"

In addition to his undergraduate degree in chemistry, Andrew earned a master's in policy, planning, and management. He acknowledges that his upbringing created opportunities that others may not have. "My recovery and sobriety didn't come easily, nor did they happen by accident. I worked hard, but I had a network and was literally afforded the space and given the opportunities to change. I had support, advocates, and mentors. I knew who I could go to without judgment. I had a team, a family, who said, 'OK, this is happening, where do we go from here? What's next, what's next, what's next? We're in this together.' Things were not done for me, and certainly not done at me. I had to do the things, but they were done with me."

Ten years into his recovery, Andrew is chief executive officer of Coatings2Go, a small company owned by his mother that produces specialized plastic coatings for medical devices.

Education can be an essential building block of recovery. It can facilitate a shift from a life centered around drugs to a life focused on self-exploration, growth, accomplishment, and contributing to the community. Some people return to an interrupted high school or college education or start fresh with new vocational and educational opportunities and goals. Others pursue learning through new relationships, reading, and trying new things. For young adults especially, formal education may be part of the stabilization stage of early recovery when they practice newly acquired skills like goal setting and accountability and figure out their next steps in the work world.

School isn't for everybody. For people who didn't fit in socially or academically, had a disruptive or violent home life, or had unaddressed learning difficulties or mental health problems, the middle or high school experience may have been bad or even traumatizing. For some people, schools were metrics of worthiness, and they feel as if they didn't measure up. It's easy to understand why they choose a recovery path that doesn't include formal education. But education doesn't just mean school. Lifelong learning is for everyone. As Andrew says, "For me, education was important, but not just education in school. A good education gives you short-term security, but more generally, recovery is a path of discovery, of learning and searching for knowledge, and that's what leads to long-term stability."

Recovery Programs

Collegiate Recovery Programs[2]
Alcohol and other drug use, including study drugs like Ritalin and Adderall and drugs produced in illegal labs and available online, is rampant on most college and university campuses in the United States, making them difficult or unsafe places for the estimated 600,000 college students in recovery.[3] Most colleges and universities provide individual or group counseling on campus or links to off-site services to address the clinical aspects of substance use disorder. These are important, but they lack the connection and solidarity that form when students in recovery come together. This peer support is one crucial element in making sure students in recovery stay in school and thrive. That's why some schools offer Collegiate Recovery Programs (CRPs) to help students sustain their recovery as they earn their degrees.

According to the Association of Recovery in Higher Education, there are currently more than 140 CRPs in the United States.[4] Each is different and reflects the college or university culture in which it operates, but they share some common characteristics. College leadership and administrators commit to creating an environment that supports recovery within the campus culture. They send a strong signal to students that they are serious about the program by providing and maintaining funding for dedicated staff and space for meetings and socializing. CRPs promote abstinence-based recovery and help students gain recovery capital in several ways. They fund substance-free activities, and some support substance-free dorms. Most hold some sort of back-to-school social event for returning and new students, and they also have "recovery graduations"—in addition to traditional graduation ceremonies—for students in the program. They support student-led initiatives like training for faculty and student leaders on addiction, recovery, and reducing stigma. Many CRPs offer leadership-development programs, opportunities for volunteering and advocacy, and links to the broader recovery community.

Finding peer support is the No. 1 reason students choose to participate in CRPs.[5] Having money troubles, being away from home and dealing with loneliness, sorting out relationship problems, meeting deadlines, and setting educational and career goals can create stress when students are learning how to cope without substances. Students I've talked with say that being part of the CRP helped them deal with stress that could lead to relapses.

FINANCIAL AID FOR PEOPLE IN RECOVERY

Scholarships and student loans are available for most college students to help pay for tuition, books, and other expenses. Eligibility for some federal aid, though, may be limited if you have any past drug convictions. It's worth asking the financial aid officer at the institution you're interested in attending for more information. Make sure to double-check information on eligibility at Federal Student Aid at www.studentaid. gov or contact your congressional representative, because eligibility requirements change. Local recovery community centers also may have helpful information.

Even if you're ineligible for federal aid, you should complete the Free Application for Federal Student Aid (FAFSA) form. That's the form the federal government uses to assess financial need. Most schools use FAFSA information to award other types of aid, including scholarships from private foundations, and you might be eligible for some of those funds.

Like the ROCC at USM, most CRPs in the United States start with a small group of students in recovery coming together for a weekly recovery support meeting, often in a classroom or shared meeting space. They grow as more students join, and eventually, the school administration provides financial support. Strong participation by substance use counselors experienced in identifying students at risk, providing counseling, and inviting students to be part of the CRP allows the program to be integrated into campus mental health programs. Large universities, small colleges, and community colleges can create Collegiate Recovery Programs. Depending on the size of the school, a CRP can serve as few as five students to more than ten. Many programs include people in recovery from mental health issues and process addictions like gambling and food addictions.[6]

CRPs are grounded in recovery research on adults showing the effectiveness of recovery housing, peer supports, access to continuing treatment and care, and mutual help groups. It makes sense that they would contribute to improved student health and increased recovery capital, but there's little research to tell us what about CRPs is the most effective. Studies show that students participating in CRPs have good academic outcomes and can sustain their recovery. On average, they have higher grade point averages and higher graduation rates than the general student population. Those who participate in CRPs may reduce their recovery-relapse cycle by fifteen years.[7, 8, 9]

Recovery High Schools

The high school years can be difficult, and young people recovering from substance use disorders have additional challenges finding their place in the world. The mainstream high school scene may be unsafe due to the presence of drugs and alcohol and a toxic social environment. No matter how helpful parents, friends, teachers, and guidance counselors try to be, sometimes a typical high school just isn't the right place for a student recovering from a substance use disorder. Recovery high schools help students build recovery capital by providing a safe environment that focuses on abstinence and education, with hands-on support from teachers and substance use counselors. Students often attend recovery high schools after treatment, giving them a fresh start with new peers and a substance-free environment.

Ideally, recovery high schools are part of the continuum of care. Treatment facilities, family members, health care providers, and the courts can make a referral with the assurance that the young person will continue to receive individual and group counseling, peer support, and opportunities for community connection and growth as well as a solid education. Recovery high schools may further support students by offering family education and counseling as well. Most are small schools with enrollments of five to seventy students, with individualized education programs that generally follow the same high school curriculum as an affiliated public or private school. Recovery high schools meet state requirements for awarding a secondary school diploma.

Like Collegiate Recovery Programs, recovery high schools are based on recovery research on adults that identifies the importance of peer support and a continuum of care. Research on adolescent recovery is emerging, and the role of education is one area of research.[10] Unfortunately, there are few recovery high schools in the United States. While there's no formal system for keeping track, the Association of Recovery Schools lists forty-three schools in twenty states.[11] There is little research on the effectiveness of recovery high schools, but what there is indicates that they are successful in maintaining the therapeutic benefits of clinical treatment and helping students attain similar levels of academic growth—even after experiencing a relapse—compared with their peers who aren't in recovery. In addition, students in recovery high schools for at least six months show a significant reduction in substance use and absenteeism.[12, 13, 14]

What Can Allies Do?

Education can be a vital part of building a new life in recovery. Formal education through online and in-person programs for credit is important for many young people. In addition, some colleges and universities support students in recovery through formal Collegiate Recovery Programs, and others create links with recovery support services in the surrounding community. Recovery high schools are available in some areas of the United States, but their number and enrollments are limited.

For Family Members and Friends

- If your loved one is interested in a recovery high school, go to the Association of Recovery Schools to learn more and find out if there's a recovery high school in your area: https://recoveryschools.org/find-a-school/.

- If your loved one doesn't know about CRPs or knows about them and is interested in a college with recovery support services on campus or in the surrounding community, ask if they would like you to help research the possibilities of Collegiate Recovery Programs that follow the standards and recommendations of the Association of Recovery in Higher Education. Offer to visit the campus and check out services in the community with them to help them learn more and feel comfortable in new recovery settings.

- If finances are a barrier to college, ask if your loved one would consider starting at a community college that offers courses that count toward a four-year degree. Ask if they would like you to contact financial aid officers for more information about specific opportunities and help fill out the Free Application for Federal Student Aid (FAFSA) form. Even if your loved one isn't eligible for federal aid, be sure they fill it out, so the institution has all of the financial information it needs to assign other forms of aid.

- Going back to school or starting a new educational path can be challenging and frightening for people who haven't had good experiences in high school or college. Find ways to be encouraging and supportive. If your loved one or friend is going to college and living at home, ask if you can help by finding substance-free activities on campus or in the community and offer to go along. If they are living on campus, learn about the resources available to support their recovery, including mental health counseling and peer groups. Offer to attend recovery-related events on campus or in the community with them.

For Everyone

- Watch *Generation Found,* a film by Jeff Reilly and Greg Williams about how community members came together to build a peer-driven youth and family recovery community in Houston that includes a system of treatment centers, recovery high schools, alternative peer groups, and Collegiate Recovery Programs.

- Some people pick up skills like time management, delayed satisfaction, and persistence when they're young, and others don't. If having these "soft skills" seems obvious to you, it's not to everyone. It's not a good idea to assume that, for example, "everyone knows that a good education leads to good employment" or "if you put in the work now, it will pay off later." If you know people in early recovery who are struggling to make sense of the long-term benefits of education, ask if they'd like you to help them think through what they may be able to accomplish later if they take time now to go to school and stay there. You may also want to ask questions like, "What do you think you'd like to be doing five years from now?" and help them think about how to get there.

- Be aware that you may be a model for people in recovery, whether or not you know it. If you've had success with your education and career path, be sure to support their ideas for their future, even if it's not the path you followed or you don't feel it's in their best interest. If they ask, share your successes and challenges.

For High School Teachers and Guidance Counselors

- Learn about Collegiate Recovery Programs in colleges and universities that your students may attend. Then when a junior or senior in your school who is in recovery or interested in trying recovery is considering a community college or four-year college program, you'll be ready to offer them information that may help them decide which college to attend.

- Learn about recovery high schools at the Association of Recovery Schools to see if there is one nearby where you can refer students in recovery. If you have the interest and motivation, you might consider starting a recovery high school where you live: https://recovery-schools.org/find-a-school/.

For College Administrators

- Ask students in recovery to participate in wellness and housing committees.

- Learn about addiction and recovery, the recovery resources in your area, and what your institution can do to support students in recovery. Learn about CRPs to see if one might be a good fit for your student body. Reach out to administrators and staff at established CRPs for more information. They can share their policies and procedures for developing a CRP.

- If students in recovery are interested in forming a program, ask how you can support them, and be ready to act. One challenge many student groups face initially is finding a space that is consistently available for meetings. Offer a classroom or other private room that students can use for 12-step meetings and other recovery support meetings.

- Learn about recovery high schools where your students typically live. Then reach out to see if they're interested in a partnership for their graduating seniors.

19

A NOTE ON FULFILLMENT

ERIK, A THIRTYSOMETHING in recovery for more than fifteen years from heroin addiction, is a tattoo artist. He says tattooing replaces the compulsion to use drugs. Now he "gets in the flow" when he tattoos.

"I started my tattoo apprenticeship seven years after I finished rehab," Erik says. "I spent those seven years making this huge effort to have a normal life. I worked in a group home [for people with disabilities] for five years, I was on Suboxone for 3.5 years, and I was in a good relationship. My girlfriend played a huge role. She really saved my life. Our relationship was so stable. She was super patient and understanding. I always felt safe with her."

But then he started to feel "stuck."

"I liked my work, giving hands-on care to clients, but I hit a ceiling. I could go into management at the group home, and then I'd be overworked and not doing the fun part of the job. I'd have all of this money and little time," so eventually he decided to switch gears and become a tattoo artist.

"There were two layers to my recovery," Erik explains. "First, I entered the Suboxone world and got a job I enjoyed. Tapering off Suboxone was really difficult because I felt things again, and then I had to work on dealing with my feelings. That's when I learned the importance of discovering what I liked, of having a goal, taking steps to achieve that goal, then reassess and making new goals. Part of being an addict is not going anywhere, so for me, there's some stability in setting goals."

Erik chose a nonconventional path after that. "For me, the idea of getting sober, throwing away all the bad things, doing what you're supposed to do, and then getting married and having kids flies in the face of following your dreams—unless it's always been your dream to have a family. For me, just fulfilling a role didn't work. When I'm tattooing, I'm doing art. I'm not fulfilling any roles.

"Failure and shame are a big part of being an addict," Erik explains. "Reframe that. Explore what you like and learn to accept failure. With art, you can make something and just tear it up if you don't like it. You can apply that to anything. If you're enjoying doing something, there's no such thing as failure. Or you can enjoy it and fail. As you do this—practice—you learn that these aren't failures at all; they're just learning. If I do the best tattoo that I can possibly do, then I go home that night and know it's enough. So, there's a connection between doing something right and my own value."

Erik has some advice for people just starting out in recovery. "Explore and discover things you like. Depending on when you started using, you might not know what you like at all. Then you start to learn that life can be cool without drugs. It's not just drudgery. It's not just following all these rules you were trying to avoid in the first place. Life can be fun, and you can have highs in life that are directly derived from the things you are doing. You can make experiences to get high. You can choose."

Education and employment are building blocks of recovery that can support a new life trajectory that includes joy and fulfillment. Like Erik, people who began using drugs or alcohol early in life may not have had a chance to figure out what they enjoy or where they find meaning, or maybe they had hobbies and friends that they turned away from when their drug use intensified. The skills and strategies learned in counseling or from peers and the job skills and intellectual development gained in school are important, but for many they're not sufficient for happiness in recovery. When people in recovery find a sense of purpose—what motivates them, what they're passionate about and gives them satisfaction at the end of the day—they turn away from drugs and alcohol to fill their internal void.

Some people in recovery find deep meaning and fulfillment in reaching out to people in distress in addiction either through volunteer work or as professional substance use counselors. Many people in recovery find deep joy in their families, especially their children. Others, like Erik, find fulfillment in a nontraditional path that includes creative expression. People in recovery don't have a monopoly on this self-actualization, on becoming their best selves, of course. But after the shame and degradation of addiction, the feeling of finding purpose in life is often more intense and fills people with more satisfaction than it does for the rest of us.

This doesn't mean that the aftereffects of trauma or other reasons people started to use in the first place are gone, but their lives take on new meaning. Nor does it mean that everyone in recovery reaches lofty heights of joy and fulfillment, just as not everyone in the general population has experiences of great achievement and purpose. People who share their recovery stories of personal fulfillment and purpose publicly are a minority of people in recovery, and they're not representative of others in recovery. Many people in recovery just want to get on with their lives privately. As Carolyn says, "We're just ordinary people living ordinary lives." Nonetheless, many recovery narratives that reflect this joy and sense of purpose in life are full of hope for people who are struggling in addiction and inspiring for all of us.

SECTION 7
The Pillars of Recovery: Community

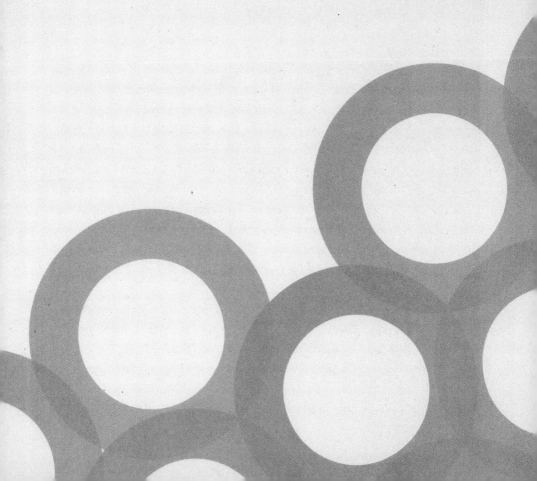

20

RECOVERY COMMUNITY
ORGANIZATIONS AND
PEER SUPPORT

WITH HER INTENSE energy, tireless dedication to women in recovery, and straight talk, Honesty Liller is a force of nature. She's married with two children, runs a small business with her husband, and recently completed a book about her experiences in addiction and recovery. She's also the CEO of the McShin Foundation, a recovery community organization (RCO) in Richmond, Virginia. She explains how she got there. "I started using drugs and alcohol when I was eleven years old, and I used for fourteen years. I used everything. And me being named Honesty? That's a laugh. I was the biggest, sneakiest liar there was during that time!" She was in and out of detox and treatment for years, and finally, her family had had enough. Her stepmother knew the director of the McShin Foundation, and she pleaded with Honesty to give the place a try. "Just do this one thing and see if it works. Just do this one last thing," she said.

"May 27, 2007, was the miracle day," Honesty says. John Shinholser, director of McShin, connected Honesty with a physician who prescribed Suboxone on a Sunday. "That doctor gave me the pill and sat with me for a few hours while it took effect. For $100, he took his Sunday and sat with me all afternoon," she says. "That was the first part of the miracle." She moved into one of McShin's three recovery residences the next day and lived there for five months. "My plan was to stay at

the house a few days to detox and then go back to my boyfriend and live together in recovery, but I stayed in the house. Something happened there! The other part of the miracle was the peer-to-peer connection, seeing other people who had been through what I'd been through and seeing them in their recovery. Opioid detox and the peer-to-peer connection saved my life."

That was during the early days of the McShin Foundation, when the organiza- tion was in two small offices in a church building. She didn't have any money for the bed fees at the recovery residence, so she worked for the foundation, and John eventually hired her as a peer coordinator. A few years later, she was promoted to CEO. Now the organization takes up three floors of that same building, runs eleven recovery residences, holds a family night to educate and support families, and runs 12-step and support group meetings. McShin hosts social events every month like dances and nature walks and runs local jail and prison programs. "We do out-of-the- box stuff," Honesty explains, "to fill voids in the community.

"I'm proud of what I've become. I'm 98 percent completely a different human since I lived here and started working here," Honesty says. "Sure, I'm the CEO, and that's great, but the real work is diving in with the women who come here and saying, 'I was you.' For example, a woman came in here, and she was pregnant. She didn't know the father, she was angry, she was on scholarship, and she didn't want to be here. I shared my experience of being pregnant, what it was like, and how I felt. She ended up staying, and then she worked here for a while. We all adopted her son, a little McShin sidekick! It's that 'been there, done that in addiction and recovery' that sets us apart. I can get real with a woman here and help her."

The McShin Foundation is one of more than one hundred recovery community organizations (RCOs) in the United States. Historically, profes- sional treatment and mutual aid groups were the two main types of assis- tance available to people on their recovery journey. In the 1970s, recovery residences were a critical addition for people who needed help after treat- ment or incarceration and before returning to family or independent living. Now RCOs, recovery community centers (RCCs), and peer recovery support services (PRSS) are on the list of recovery support services, especially for people in the first years of recovery.

John Shinholser, a cofounder of McShin, explains how it works: "We're boots on the ground, dealing with the day in and day out needs of the com- munity. We try to stay in sync with what's happening nationally [in recovery support services, research, funding, and advocacy], but we don't wait around for permission to do anything. We're doers, man. We innovate. We respond to the needs of our people the minute they call or walk in the door. We connect to them as peers, and we link them to treatment, housing, food, clothing, whatever they need at that moment. We want to be there for somebody when the hand of recovery reaches up. Without that, you've got nothing."

RCO OR RCC?

The terms "recovery community center" and "recovery community organization" are sometimes used interchangeably, but they're not the same. Both are independent, nonprofit organizations governed by people in recovery and family members, friends, and allies. RCCs are typically smaller than RCOs and function locally to provide direct peer support services, social and recreational opportunities, links to local services, and community education. RCOs often function at the regional or state level and focus on public education and awareness, mobilizing resources, and advocating for policies that support recovery. Some RCOs are RCCs, like the McShin Foundation, and provide direct peer support services in local communities. Both RCOs and RCCs develop recovery leaders and are the "voice of recovery" in their communities and states.[1, 2, 3]

RCO best practices, developed by Faces and Voices of Recovery, a national recovery advocacy organization, is available at https://faces andvoicesofrecovery.org/arco/rco-best-practices/.

Recovery Community Centers

The idea of a place where people in recovery can meet and socialize isn't new. Alcoholics Anonymous "clubhouses" started in the 1940s, and now there are hundreds of them across the United States. These are private clubs funded by member dues that support the 12-step pathway to recovery. In addition to having 12-step meetings, AA clubhouses also host dinners, dances, and other social gatherings.

Recovery community centers, in contrast, are free to anyone and support all recovery pathways. RCCs are located within the community they serve: in densely populated urban areas with large numbers of marginalized members, in more well-off suburbs, as well as in small towns with few members and powerful social connections that work in favor of building community recovery capital. They're not drop-in centers or treatment agencies. Instead, they're recovery sanctuaries that provide recovery coaching, telephone support, skill development like relapse prevention, and naloxone trainings (to reverse opioid overdoses). RCCs are safe spaces with access to computers and the internet, links to employment and job training opportunities, volunteer opportunities in the community, and recovery housing. They host support group meetings, including 12-step meetings. They're hubs of substance-free recreational and social events, yoga and meditation groups, recovery art shows, and places where people can go for support. They come in all sizes, with some having just a few visitors per month and others having thousands. Some are grassroots operations with few resources, and others are well-funded setups with sophisticated social media outreach and technology to track visits using scannable membership cards.

RCCs reflect the community they serve, including racial and sexual diversity. That said, people in marginalized communities and rural areas may find themselves in "recovery deserts" with no RCC or other recovery support services. People of color and the LGBTQIA+ community are underrepresented in most recovery communities and may not find the services they want in recovery community centers. Cultural and language differences, including among immigrants, create barriers to integrating into the mainstream recovery community. Some RCCs address these challenges by offering meetings (usually 12-step meetings) in different languages in areas where English is the dominant language. Others recognize that not everyone wants to come to the RCC building and reach out to learn what they can do to support recovery outside the RCC.

Most RCCs link people to basic necessities like clothing and food and provide medical services on site like HIV testing and smoking cessation. Some RCCs operate recovery residences, some give onsite counseling, and a few provide access to Suboxone. Residential treatment centers have hopped on the recovery bandwagon and now call themselves "recovery centers," but they're nothing like

RCCs. What sets recovery community centers and recovery community organizations apart is that they are run by and for people in recovery. In the words of one member, "RCCs are a place where the recovery community welcomes you when you're ready to come home."

RCCs are essential for some people in the early weeks and months of recovery as a place to develop new networks, go to meetings, and get connected with critical resources like recovery housing. Sometimes they're just a "place to go" when there's no place else. RCCs are helpful for people in long-term recovery, too. Long after the initial recovery journey starts, many people experience challenges in employment, education, and family and social relations.[4] RCCs link them to job openings, educational opportunities, and other resources that may help.

RCCs are places where families can reconnect after years of addiction. As Honesty from the McShin Foundation says, "As people who are using drugs, we harm our families because they're the easiest to harm. We steal. We lie. So, it's important to heal the families because most people end up going back to their families. Maybe they don't live with them, but they're family. No matter what, your family is your family." In addition to providing education, support groups, and information on treatment, recovery residences, and other services, RCCs provide family members opportunities to meet with their peers. In family groups or one-on-one, they learn from each other how to "be there" for the people they love even when that's difficult, where the best recovery support services are, and how to take care of themselves when the going gets tough.

The team of paid staff and volunteers who operate RCCs are often in recovery. Most RCCs receive state or federal funding in addition to private funding from local organizations and foundations. The peer support of paid staff and recovery coaches, volunteers, and unstructured member-to-member relationships form the core of RCCs.

Research

Theoretical explanations of what makes recovery community organizations successful sound dreary compared with John's description of McShin. "McShin was started around a campfire at a 12-step campout. The idea, the vision came: addicts sharing and caring in the way they do. That was a Saturday night, and Monday morning, the LLC was assigned. Wednesday, the office was open. Just like that. No business plan, no system. Just vision, passion, and a little bit of compulsion." John's wife, Carol McDaid, a well-known recovery advocate, knew about addiction and recovery policy issues at the national level, and John was an entrepreneur. *"We started McShin with a combination of the old-timer recovery spirit, the obvious need to give what had been given to us, the knowledge that this [recovery support services] was an emerging industry, and the desire to be a pioneer in this industry in the twenty-first century.*

"From there, the beacon of hope started to shine bright. And, of course, that beacon sucks in the hopeless. And when you combine a vision of hope with hopelessness, and when the hope dealer understands the need to empower the hopeless to take ownership of the process, what you're seeing today [the McShin Foundation] is the result of that."

Emerging evidence indicates that recovery community centers' role in the continuum of recovery supports is linking people to resources that increase their recovery capital. A study of RCCs in the northeastern part of the United States found that most people who frequented RCCs were white and between the ages of twenty-five and fifty-nine. Most had fallen on hard times because of their addiction, and they had lower incomes and education levels than their peers in the general public. Many were unemployed, and many were involved with the criminal justice system. Most people had some co-occurring mental health condition and were in recovery from alcohol or opioids; most had regularly used multiple substances.[5]

Interestingly, research shows that people who visit RCCs gain more recovery capital but not more social support than people who don't. It's likely that RCC members already have social support from 12-step meetings and recovery residences. The other RCC services, like links to employment and other opportunities to boost recovery capital, are more directly related to being at the RCC.[6]

The Importance of Peers

Peers are at the heart of recovery community centers, where people in recovery can meet other people in recovery and move away from their drug-using friends. Peers help with problem solving and provide role models, especially for people in early recovery. Perhaps most important, though, is the empathy and nonjudgmental support that people share with one another.

Most people I talked with made a point of setting peers apart from professional counselors and therapists they'd seen. A refrain in nearly all of the interviews mirrored one young man's comment, "The care I've received from professional providers has been dwarfed by the care I've received from fellow people in recovery." Honesty, the CEO of the McShin Foundation, echoed this comment. "After years of seeing professionals—people who were trying to help me—I couldn't connect with anyone until I lived at McShin. They took me in, and they helped me like no one else could."

Informal peer support happens everywhere, any time people in recovery come together. More formal support, usually in the form of a trained recovery coach, is an up-and-coming recovery support service. One definition of peer recovery support services (PRSS) is the "process of giving and receiving nonprofessional, nonclinical assistance to achieve long-term recovery from substance use disorder."[7] Peers embody the hope of recovery. They support others along their recovery journey and help build recovery capital by increasing skills, addressing specific needs people face, and expanding social networks in the recovery community. PRSS don't give advice, diagnose, or provide therapy.[8]

Most coaches receive three to four days of formal training in recovery pathways, self-reflection to understand personal biases, active listening and communication skills, stages of change and stages of recovery, stigma, power and privilege, boundary issues, self-care, crisis intervention, sexual harassment, recovery capital, and developing a recovery wellness plan. Overall, the goal is to learn how to be empathetic and nonjudgmental and treat people as resources in their own recovery.[9] Some states have certification requirements for recovery coaches.

RCCs often train and hire recovery coaches to provide one-on-one coaching sessions, group sessions, and telephone support and contribute to the culture of nonjudgmental communication at the center. Addiction treatment centers now hire recovery coaches to bridge treatment and recovery support services in the community. Jails, prisons, faith organizations, recovery residences, probation and parole programs, drug courts, and other institutions also engage with recovery coaches. Health care organizations like primary care physicians and hospital emergency rooms hire coaches to integrate formal care with peer support and link people with resources outside the health care setting. Depending on the organization, recovery coaches may be outreach workers, part of the clinical team, or work independently.

As these organizations expand their workforce to include recovery coaching, new issues arise. Recovery coach training is essential, but should coaches be credentialed so they meet specific standards? In a setting outside a recovery community center, who supervises them? Should their supervisors have lived experience? What are the roles and responsibilities of coaches in hospitals, treatment facilities, prisons, and other settings? How do coaches deal with confidentiality when they're part of a treatment team? Should they share information learned in coaching sessions? If coaches are paid, how does their pay align with that of the rest of the behavioral health workforce? What should public and private insurance reimbursement for coaching services be? These are some of the many questions that will be answered as recovery coaching expands in multiple settings.

Reality Check is a small recovery community center in south-central New Hampshire that has started to answer some of these questions. Mary Drew, a woman in recovery, started Reality Check at her kitchen table shortly after entering recovery, driven by a passion for helping her community solve its addiction and overdose problems. Now Reality Check is part of the statewide recovery network in New Hampshire and is listed in the Recovery Hub, a project of the New Hampshire government to provide residents reliable information and recovery support services across the state.[10] Mary and her staff work in a mixed-use building and provide space for 12-step meetings, support groups, and one-on-one counseling sessions. They recently partnered with a small local hospital to develop a pilot recovery coaching program in the emergency room, and it expanded to be hospital-wide and includes coverage for its four affiliate offices. Reality Check staff created a handbook for recovery coaches, a training video for hospital staff, and a protocol for linking patients with coaches. The area is extremely rural, and the hospital can't support a paid recovery coach on staff, so instead, coaches trained through Reality Check receive a small stipend when they are on-call for twelve-hour shifts and a gas card if they are dispatched. Coaches meet monthly for supervision with a master's trained alcohol and drug counselor and have additional group supervision with the coach coordinator at Reality Check. "We're always looking for critical points of intervention where we can better impact the epidemic, while increasing awareness around resources and sharing success stories," Mary says. "The recovery coach program and our partnership with the hospital are one of those interventions. It's one way we keep recovery central and strong in our area, as well as raising the voice of recovery in the state."

Research

Research on formal peer recovery support services is emerging, and researchers are working on determining what is effective about the peer relationship. Generally, evidence indicates that formal peer recovery supports have a positive effect on people receiving services but doesn't tell us which approaches and types of support work best, the amount and intensity of the peer intervention, the skill level of the peer, the setting where the service is delivered, and the effectiveness in different populations.[11, 12] In other words, it seems as if peer recovery support services are effective, but we're not sure why or how.

One report on peer recovery support services in Philadelphia's recovery-focused behavioral health care system shows enhanced abstinence, increases in employment, educational involvement, housing stability, and parental custody of children.[13] Many research projects are underway to understand whether embedding recovery coaches in health care organizations, treatment agencies, jails, prisons, drug courts, and other organizations results in better outcomes for people in recovery. Many of those projects consider not just the effectiveness of coaching on recovery outcomes but also the cost-effectiveness of using recovery coaches.

Who Can Become a Coach?

Most recovery coaches are people in recovery, but family members, community members, and other allies are trained in some parts of the country. Local attitudes prevail, and some people argue that only people in recovery can be good coaches. Others believe that being caring, compassionate, and open-minded are the most critical requirements for being an effective coach. The debate here goes back to being an authentic peer. Can you do that if you don't have the lived experience of recovery? Opinions differ.

The Connecticut Community for Addiction Recovery is one of the organizations that believes that you can be a family member, friend, or ally who isn't in recovery and be an excellent coach. Phil Valentine, executive director and a man in long-term recovery, explains: "What is the essence of the 'lived experience' in recovery we hear so much about? It helps people connect. But if you're lit up, if your fire is stoked internally, it's really just the ability to love and care and sit with somebody and have your spirit warm theirs. It's a spiritual connection. The recovery community doesn't have a monopoly on this. If you have the right heart for coaching and support, if you have the 'mojo,' it doesn't matter whether you're in recovery or not.

"If you can listen, ask good questions, discover and manage your own 'stuff,' if you can treat people like a resource in their own recovery, then you can become a recovery coach.

"You have to meet people 'where they're at,'" Phil says. "That means whether they're taking methadone and drinking on weekends, using marijuana, on medication-assisted treatment, or none of those, you meet them there even though this might challenge your own beliefs about the definition of recovery. So, recovery coaches, when they're doing it right, are asking, 'What does recovery mean to you?' and listening to the answer."

What Can Allies Do?

For Everyone

- Learn about the recovery community centers in your area and the services they offer. If they hold public events like recovery rallies or community meetings, try to attend and bring a friend!

- RCCs are first and foremost created by and for the recovery community. If there's an effort to start an RCC in your town or city and you like the idea of a place for people in recovery to go for support, become a part of it. But realize that if there's no energy in the recovery community for a center, it's not appropriate to start one "for them."

- RCCs serve people in all stages of recovery, and some of them need necessities like clothing, women's products, and toiletries. For those that help women with children, donations of baby items, including diapers, are welcome. Before donating, check with staff at the center to ask what they need most.

- If you live in an area where community members can become recovery coaches, explore options for training, usually through a recovery community center.

- Ask about being a volunteer or being a community member on the board. RCCs can always use more hands to help at events. They can benefit from donated legal, accounting, administrative, cleaning, and maintenance services. Community members serving on the board can link the RCC to other organizations and help with fundraising.

For Community Organizations

- Work with the local RCC to find ways to offer childcare during meetings at the center and daycare while parents are at work if the RCC has identified that as a need.

- Reach out to your local RCC and offer life skills that are part of your existing work—classes on cooking, money management, food shopping on a budget, or time management for single parents, if the RCC has identified that as a need.

For Health Care Providers

- Visit your local RCCs to learn about the peer recovery support services they offer and link your patients in recovery to them.

- If you're interested in a recovery coach program at your practice or hospital, reach out to the local RCC to find out what they can offer as a partner. Check to see if your state has a certification or licensing requirement for coaches.

SECTION 8
Recovery Advocacy

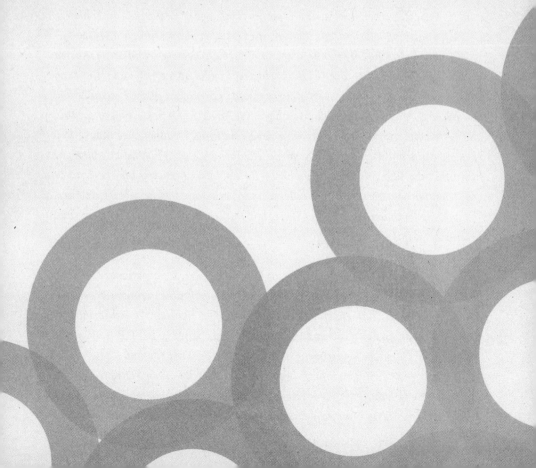

21

ADVOCACY

TOM CODERRE IS in long-term recovery and is well known in the recovery community. He introduces himself with the positive language of recovery: "I am a man in
long-term recovery, which means I haven't used drugs or alcohol since May 15, 2003."

Tom had been a Rhode Island state senator for eight years when his drug use sent
his life careening off the rails. "I lost everything I cared about," he says. "I lost my
position in the state Senate. I lost a job in a large nonprofit. I pushed away family
and friends." After being kicked out of his house, arrested for possession of cocaine,
and undergoing six months of court-ordered residential treatment, he moved to a
recovery residence in Providence, near his childhood home. While he was there, he
heard that the Rhode Island Communities for Addiction Recovery Efforts, a recovery community organization, was holding a legislative day to advocate for recovery.
"I signed up to volunteer then and there, and that changed everything," Tom says.
"That started my journey in policy work." ·

Soon after the legislative day, Tom attended a media and messaging training
session conducted by Faces and Voices of Recovery (FAVOR), a national advocacy
organization, where attendees learned how to talk about their recovery experience
in a positive light. "That was transformational for me," Tom says. "I was looking for
words to talk about my recovery to the general public, and the FAVOR training did
that." He chose to make his recovery story about personal redemption.

He took a job as national field director of FAVOR's Recovery Voices Count initiative during the 2008 election season. "That was before candidates were willing
to talk about recovery," Tom explains. "We picked ten battleground states, did some

nonpartisan civic engagement, voter registration and get-out-the-vote activities. We *used the election as a platform to organize the recovery community to advocate for* *themselves."*

Tom returned to the Rhode Island Senate as chief of staff for the Senate president for six years and went on to become chief of staff for the Substance Abuse and Mental Health Services Administration. There, he led the research and publication of Facing Addiction in America: The Surgeon General's Report on Alcohol, Drugs, and Health. He also fought for passage of the 21st Century Cures Act in 2016, which designated $1 billion in grants for states to fight the opioid epidemic. This was the first time Congress had made significant federal funding available for treatment of opioid use disorder, a testimony to recovery advocacy efforts across the country.

"I've been on the front lines and had a front-row seat to what has been happening for years," Tom says. "We have a much bigger platform today because of the opioid crisis. We should use it! People are dying from opioids right now, and that is what is getting the attention. But we have an addiction crisis. And we have a mental health crisis. We have too many deaths from alcohol, opioids, suicide," he says passionately. "Thank God the media and others have started paying attention. If it's opioids that got them to pay attention, let's use that.

"There are things that people in our community need, and it's time that we make sure they have them. We need to own this, take back what is rightfully ours, and advocate for those things. The No. 1 advocacy goal should be building recovery support services, including in rural areas. We need recovery support services extended beyond or instead of treatment, up to five years after treatment. That means recovery coaching and other peer support, virtual recovery resources, recovery housing. We should be advocating for building people's health care for those five years, their home for those five years, their purpose (usually connection to a job, which is where people find purpose), and we should connect them back to the community so that they are full, active citizens. That's because, after five years of recovery, the chance of remission returns to 15 percent, and that's what other chronic diseases use as a success marker. These are the things that the recovery community should be working on."

Tom pauses and says thoughtfully, "All of these things are the blessings of recovery, but that's not everything. I got to be a son to my father, and I got to be with my mom to help her when my dad passed."

Recovery advocacy takes place in the Oval Office, the halls of Congress and state legislatures, and at town and city council meetings. It also happens in community task forces, coalitions, boardrooms, and committees. We use positive stories of recovery like Tom's and family stories of renewal to change hearts and minds about people in recovery. We use those stories, backed up by research and data, to ask decision makers to fund evidence-based recovery support services. There's a place for your voice, where you can bring your energy, ideas, and connections to bear on increasing recovery capital and supporting people in recovery in your community.

What Is Advocacy?

Advocacy is a general term that can mean personal advocacy—speaking up for yourself or someone else—or working to change a significant social problem like environmental degradation or homelessness. Some people are professional advocates, and others are laypeople who show up and speak up from time to time. Many advocates have personal experiences with their topic, and others are people who see an injustice—like the stigma, discrimination, and lack of appropriate services for people in recovery—and want to do something about it. People in recovery and their families often have a passion to "give back." Friends and family who have lost people they love to overdoses want to make sure other families are spared the pain they've endured.

There are quite a few formal definitions of advocacy, but I like this simple one: *Advocacy is getting other people to do what you want them to do so you get what you want.*

Let's break that down. First, it's important to figure out who "you" is. If you're working in your neighborhood or town, maybe "you" is the people who live there, or "you" is family members impacted by addiction. After you know who "you" is, figure out what you want. Perhaps you want a safe place for people to live in early recovery. It's essential to be specific so that you can figure out what needs to change, so you get what you want. That will determine who can help you.

In our example of safe housing for people in early recovery, advocacy will look something like this:

1. Find out who "you" is by looking for other people who agree there's a need for recovery housing in your neighborhood or town. People in recovery, other families impacted by addiction, housing and homeless coalitions and advocates, health care providers,

and local decision makers like council members or mayors are all possibilities. It's usually best to connect with an established group doing related work to save time and energy needed to bring people together and set up an organizational structure. You can bring your passion to the group, educate them about recovery, and focus on specific action steps. Individual initiatives are important, but it usually takes many community stakeholders working together to create a program that can succeed in the long run.

2. Do a little research to find out what types of recovery residences are already in your region. For example, you could approach a local recovery community center to find out what's available or ask people in recovery about local recovery houses. Looking online is especially important, too, to learn all you can about recovery housing. In this case, you'd look online at the National Alliance for Recovery Residences (NARR), find out if your state has an affiliate, and if so, contact them.

3. Figure out what other people need to do so that people in early recovery in your neighborhood or town have access to safe recovery housing. For example, you may find that recovery houses nearby typically have available openings. Your solution might be to ask social service providers, pastors, and others to open communication channels with the house operators about how to refer people to the houses.

4. If you find no recovery residences nearby, your best next step is to check in with your local housing coalition, substance use coalition, or NARR affiliate. Those entities have organizational structures in place, including staff who can help you determine the best way to get a recovery house in your area. If you're not already part of a coalition, offer to join and help focus the group's energies on recovery.

So, in this case, our advocacy steps were *getting the local housing coalition to understand the importance of recovery residences and prioritizing recovery housing in their work so that people in recovery in our community have access to recovery housing.* Notice that the original group of people didn't end up starting a recovery residence themselves. This would be putting the creation of a recovery residence in the hands of people who aren't experts in the field. The best way to get a recovery residence in place is to turn to the people who already have knowledge, organization, funding, and probably some political clout to help you get what you want.

A Note on Lobbying

People often confuse being an advocate with being a lobbyist. Lobbyists are governed by specific state and federal definitions and regulations. Generally, being a lobbyist means attempting to influence decision makers like legislators, governors, and congresspeople to vote in a certain way on a specific piece of legislation. State and federal regulations establish lobbying activities based on the amount or percentage of a person's time and income spent on influencing legislation. It usually isn't considered lobbying if your activities take only a few hours a week, you aren't paid, and your engagement with these decision makers is limited to activities like educating them on issues, introducing them to people in recovery, writing letters and emails, and testifying before legislative committees.

Conventional Advocacy to Create Policy Change

Policy change at the state or national level is the main objective for much of recovery advocacy work. Steps for this approach to change usually go something like this: Build ongoing relationships with decision makers, build a coalition of allies and organizations with a similar mission, research the situation, educate decision makers, make a specific "ask," help make it happen, and thank everyone involved. As community members, the best way to get involved in this type of advocacy is to join an existing organization working on recovery issues or, as in the case of recovery housing, related topics where you can interject recovery-specific concerns. Local and statewide recovery community organizations and statewide organizations like prisoner reentry partnerships, housing coalitions, substance use prevention coalitions, health care advocacy groups, and harm reduction coalitions are possibilities in most states. Allies may be asked to participate in strategies such as working with a legislator to propose a bill, writing letters to the editor with personal stories, creating social media posts, testifying at legislative hearings, and making one-on-one calls to legislators to educate them about the issue.

Faces and Voices of Recovery, one of the key national advocacy organizations advocating for federal policy change, has a free online toolkit specifically for recovery advocacy at www.facesandvoicesofrecovery.org/blog/publication/recovery-advocacy-toolkit/.

Electoral Advocates

These advocates work within the electoral system to educate voters about their rights, the issues, and where and when to vote. Typically, national electoral advocacy targets a few states where candidates may be recovery friendly, but they may not be frontrunners in their elections. Common strategies are grassroots organizing to "get out the vote," holding community meetings, and educating all candidates. Advocates can practice electoral advocacy for state and local elections, too.

Faces and Voices of Recovery has an ongoing Recovery Voices Count campaign for national electoral advocacy. Find information and how to be involved at www.facesandvoicesofrecovery.org/rvc/#allies.

Grassroots Organizing

If you're interested in locally driven action, grassroots organizing is the way to go. The steps are essentially the same as for conventional or electoral advocacy, but the organizing effort takes place in the community. Decision makers will usually be locally elected officials but could also be local employers or leaders of organizations who can impact change. Your base of support will be people in recovery, allies, and other community members, and your main task will be to identify them, convene them around a specific topic, and assign specific duties such as writing letters to the editor, creating social media posts, testifying at city council hearings or attending meetings with local leaders, or making calls to local decision makers.

Ryan Hampton, activist and founder of the Recovery Advocacy Project (RAP), says that "just like there are many pathways of recovery, there are many pathways of advocacy. There's room for everyone." RAP focuses on grassroots organizing and electoral advocacy so people can "make change in their own backyard." RAP provides training to local organizations, giving them the tools to think and act locally. Ryan wants to "put recovery and politics in the same sentence. Recovery isn't political," he says, "but access to recovery services and health care, private prisons, and criminal justice are political issues. We're building a community around the fact that this is an issue, a voting issue. We're holding politicians accountable." The recovery environment is different in every state, and that's where RAP puts its energy—into issues that people in each state have identified as important. Local RAP groups conduct voter registration drives, promote legislation, educate legislators, interview candidates and endorse those who are recovery friendly, create candidate "recovery report cards," and recruit advocates to testify and put pressure on legislators to change policies.

RAP has a comprehensive grassroots organizing toolkit that includes best practices for each step in the process. It's available at www.recovery voices.com/advocacy-guide.

Disruptive Advocacy

Sometimes, working through existing political channels doesn't result in the change you want. In this case, disruptive actions designed to call attention to your cause and send a blunt message to decision makers may be effective. The enormous number of overdose deaths in the recovery community has been the most prominent issue that has drawn disruptive actions. Sit-ins on the steps of city hall, marches in the streets, and staged lie-ins with people representing the numbers of deaths are common. "You Talk, We Die." "Every overdose death is a policy failure." "People who use drugs don't deserve to die." "No More Drug War." "Incarceration isn't treatment." I've seen these on placards and signs at overdose prevention vigils, harm reduction rallies, and legislative events.

Most disruptive advocacy focuses on harm reduction and ending the war on drugs. National organizations like the Drug Policy Alliance and regional organizations like the Chicago Recovery Alliance have information and resources online at www.drugpolicy.org and www.anypositivechange.org, respectively.

The Power of Stories

Adding personal stories to facts, figures, and science can be powerfully persuasive. Appealing to the human side of decision makers is a strategy used across advocacy organizations to budge the reluctant ones to change policy. National recovery advocacy organizations have developed recommendations for telling person-first recovery narratives privately to friends and family and publicly to community organizations, employers, the media, public policy makers, and others. According to Faces and Voices of Recovery, our stories should be personal, focus on the positive aspects of recovery, and talk about hopes and dreams. They should help people understand that recovery is much more than just not using drugs or alcohol—recovery is about creating a good life.[1]

From an advocacy point of view, Tom Coderre says, "The best thing we do is tell our personal stories and make it real for people and let them make their own judgment. I think that changes hearts and minds better than anything else could. And family members who tell their stories are incredibly powerful, too."

Here are some examples.

"My name is Ricardo, and I'm a person in long-term recovery. For me, that means I haven't used drugs or alcohol for over five years. I have a stable job as a carpenter that I enjoy, and my son is back in my life. I've been volunteering for the local recovery community center, where I got help and support when I needed it most. I'm taking college courses, one at a time, to learn more about owning my own business, which I want to do some day."

"My name is Monique. My son is in long-term recovery, which means he hasn't used drugs for two years. I'm so proud of him. Recovery has given me and my family stability, a new purpose, and hope for the future. I'm speaking out because long-term recovery has helped me change my life for the better, and I want to make it possible for others to do the same."

"My name is Michael, and I'm a recovery ally. I support young people in recovery who are part of our community, because they are our future. I know that recovery support services help people in early recovery find jobs and housing to achieve long-term recovery. I want them to have all of the recovery support they need so they have the same opportunities for a rich life that I have had."

RECOVERY IS PURPLE

The recovery community is diverse and includes people from all walks of life—corporate executives, frontline food service workers, veterans, doctors, construction workers, and just about any other profession or field. It includes Democrats, Republicans, Libertarians, Social Democrats, and more.

Recovery isn't a "blue" issue for Democrats or a "red" issue for Republicans. It's a "purple" issue for everyone, making national and state policy change particularly challenging. It's tempting to define ourselves by our differences rather than what unites us, ignoring the endgame of building recovery-friendly communities. Some advocates look for a policy agenda that most of us can get behind, like funding recovery support services. Others look to an issue that has less broad support like funding harm reduction services. There will be unresolvable disagreement on some issues. Because of the diversity of the recovery community and enormity of its collective issues, we need more than one advocacy agenda and more than one strategy. National and state policy change is essential, but so is changing the electoral landscape for recovery advocacy. Grassroots strategies for change in communities are vital for increasing recovery capital. Disruptive rallies and marches might not be your preference, but they have a crucial role in raising awareness about complex issues. We need multiple agendas and strategies if we're going to succeed in creating recovery-friendly communities.

The New Recovery Advocacy Movement

Being a recovery advocate means being part of a movement that has been in existence since 2001 and has gotten louder in recent years. The New Recovery Advocacy Movement started at a meeting in St. Paul, Minnesota. Fueled by growth in local recovery advocacy organizations and some funding from the federal government's Recovery Community Support Program in the 1990s, the movement picked up where previous advocacy initiatives had left off in the 1970s and gained momentum.

The foundational principles of the movement haven't changed since the 2001 meeting:

1. Addiction recovery is a living reality for individuals, families, and communities.

2. There are many (religious, spiritual, secular) pathways to recovery, and all are cause for celebration.

3. Recovery flourishes in supportive communities.

4. Recovery is a voluntary process.

5. Recovering and recovered people are part of the solution: recovery gives back what addiction has taken from individuals, families, and communities.[2]

Faces and Voices of Recovery and other national organizations are part of the New Recovery Advocacy Movement, working on policy reform. Key issues are funding recovery support services and reforming health care so that evidence-based addiction treatment can be available for anyone who needs it, when and where they need it. State affiliates of the Recovery Advocacy Project, individual state recovery coalitions like the Pennsylvania Recovery Organizations Alliance, and recovery community organizations (RCOs) are part of the New Recovery Advocacy Movement and mobilize state resources to address state policy issues such as drug sentencing reform and naloxone distribution. RCOs, recovery community centers, and local substance use coalitions are part of the movement, too. They know that addiction is a community problem with a community solution, and they focus their efforts on local solutions to promote recovery support services for specific groups in their communities. These organizations—and many others—place educating community members and decision makers about recovery and reducing stigma at the top of their list of advocacy issues.

The Advocacy Agenda

I asked fifteen leading recovery advocates and researchers about their advocacy agenda, and I got fifteen different answers. I was surprised. Tom Coderre wasn't. "People in the recovery community have a hard time articulating what they need. We've done a horrible job coming together to develop a plan, saying, 'This is what we need.' The advocacy community has been splintered, with multiple national organizations focusing on prevention and recovery, and now the harm reduction community is redefining recovery. We have work to do on this."

Advocating for recovery-friendly communities is like advocating for a solution to climate change. Many groups can have a single purpose (mitigate effects of climate change) with many strategies and agendas (such as reducing greenhouse gas emissions through public policies to promote solar and wind power and pressure on private corporations to change their use of fossil fuels). Building recovery-friendly communities requires a multipronged advocacy strategy, too.

The recovery advocacy agenda that follows is based on what I heard from advocates, researchers, and laypeople in recovery about supporting people in recovery and building recovery capital. Not surprisingly, addressing stigma and educating community members and policy makers topped the list for everyone. Making room for people following all recovery pathways in advocacy and policy work, shifting resources from acute care (treatment) to recovery support services like recovery residences, and drug policy reform were frequently mentioned as well.

Stigma and Community Education

We've seen that substance use disorder is one of the most stigmatized conditions across the globe. To address this, advocates must commit to the ongoing education of community members and decision makers. Changing the way people in our culture think about addiction isn't a one-off town hall meeting, social media campaign, or article in the newspaper. It's using all avenues of education for every segment of the community for the foreseeable future. "In a perfect world, politically and from a policy perspective, change should happen because it needs to, but it doesn't," says Philip Rutherford, chief operating officer of Faces and Voices of Recovery. Having a vocal constituency and calling out stigma are critical to making change happen. "With just those two things as policy planks, we could move the New Recovery Advocacy Movement ahead light years."

Drug Policy Reform

While the recovery community isn't united on changing drug sentencing laws or decriminalizing illegal substances, the advocates I spoke with acknowledged the harm that has been done by harsh sentences for drug possession, particularly in communities of color. "We support decriminalization without question," Rutherford says. "Part of the legacy of the recovery movement is that it formed from people whose pathway was abstinence from alcohol use, but that is no longer the case." People in recovery from illegal substance use often have criminal charges or convictions that follow them throughout their lives, impeding their ability to have stable housing, an education, and stable employment. Reducing or eliminating sentences for drug possession and creating a pathway to treatment and recovery instead—moving resources from the criminal justice system to the health care system—is an important step toward supporting individuals and communities in recovery.

Health and Health Care

Barriers to treatment, health care, and harm reduction services are significant, and recovery advocates work hard to eliminate them. William White—recovery researcher, writer, and inspiration to many—suggests a redesign of addiction treatment from acute models of care to models of sustained recovery management that use recovery as an organizing principle. Greg Williams, creator and director of the films *The Anonymous People, Generation Found,* and *Tipping the Pain Scale,* argues for health care reform to support recovery. One way to do this is to create incentives for insurance companies to improve treatment and recovery outcomes over five years, well beyond the current twenty-eight-day treatment cycle.[3] Laws and regulations governing access to medications for addiction need to be changed to increase access to treatment. Harm reductionists see funding for new and existing syringe services programs, sparsely scattered across the United States, as critical.

Home

Advocates I interviewed suggested focusing on initiatives that put housing at the center of early recovery supports. "Think of recovery housing as a launchpad for other community services people need, like job training and community mental health," says Dave Sheridan, executive director of the National Alliance for Recovery Residences. Ensuring quality recovery housing and fighting "Not In My Back Yard" attitudes ("NIMBYism") toward recovery residences are essential local advocacy tasks.

Purpose

"What does recovery look like?" Philip Rutherford asks. "In addition to stable housing, it looks like stable employment, and it looks like educational attainment." The actions laid out in chapters 17 and 18 on employment and education highlight specific steps communities can take. Applying pressure to university administrators to form Collegiate Recovery Programs and connecting people in early recovery with recovery-friendly employers are two essential actions.

Community

Phillip Valentine, executive director of the Connecticut Community for Addiction Recovery, says funding recovery community organizations (RCOs), recovery community centers (RCCs), and peer recovery support is critical. He argues for an RCO in every state, an RCC in every town, and recovery coaches at critical points of intervention like hospital emergency departments. To arrive at these goals, federal and state governments need to support building a recovery coach network through recovery coach trainings, a certification process, and a reimbursement mechanism for the deployment of recovery coaches and other peer support services.

PASSION AND POLICY

Many people who have lived through a destructive life in addiction have an immense sense of gratitude that they've found recovery, and they're passionate about the path that helped them. Sometimes they're so passionate that they want everyone to follow their path and don't consider that what worked for them doesn't work for everyone. Historically, a vocal minority of people in Alcoholics Anonymous has shaped the public dialogue about addiction and recovery with an ideology that abstinence and AA were the only path that "works," at the expense of other pathways and the science that supports them. Our addiction and recovery policies now reflect this bias through public and private payment for traditional, abstinence-based residential treatment programs developed for people with alcohol use disorder that aren't appropriate for everyone. At the same time, our policies have limited access to other types of evidence-based treatment like medications for addiction. The New Recovery Advocacy Movement is changing to keep pace with science and the needs of the recovery community. More people who have followed pathways other than 12-step programs are joining, raising their voices, and fighting for the full array of services known to help sustain recovery.

What Can Allies Do?

Community members can focus on reducing stigma and use the four pillars of recovery—Health, Home, Purpose, and Community—to guide their advocacy work. Connecting with an existing advocacy organization like a recovery community organization or substance use coalition is usually the best way to amplify your voice. It's also vital to learn advocacy tools like telling your personal story, contacting legislators, grassroots organizing, and supporting recovery-friendly candidates.

For Everyone

- Support state and federal initiatives on complex policy issues like revamping insurance regulations and coverage to support recovery for five years and changing laws and regulations to make medications for addiction easier to access. You can do this by **connecting with local and state advocacy organizations and responding to their advocacy requests.** Signing up for email and social media alerts from advocacy organizations is a great way to stay current. In addition, you may need to learn to testify before a legislative committee, tell your personal story, or write a letter to the editor.

- **Learn how to tell your story.** You can use the format proposed by Faces and Voices of Recovery. If that way of storytelling doesn't reflect your community when talking about recovery, reach out to people in recovery and ask them the best way to talk about your personal experiences. Be sure to **stay in your lane** and tell your own story, not your family member's or friend's story. If you want to add something about their recovery experience, make sure you have their permission.

- Support calls for more public funding for recovery support services by **contacting state legislators and your congressional delegation** when specific funding legislation is proposed. Advocacy organizations typically have lists of legislators and congresspeople by town or zip code to help you identify people representing you. To get their attention, remind them that they count on your vote for reelection, and you're watching their position on the legislation.

- **Be vocal about making sure people in recovery are in decision-making positions** in local and state government, university administration, employer organizations like chambers of commerce, and any state or local groups or committees addressing addiction issues.

- Many drug sentencing laws vary from state to state, and attitudes toward changing them differ considerably across the country. Community members can learn more by **reaching out to recovery advocates and state legislators.**

- If an organization working on a recovery issue—like starting a recovery community center or rallying support for a recovery residence in your neighborhood—contacts you, say "yes!" **Find a way to participate that makes sense to you.** As a visible ally, you help send a message that recovery is important to the community, not just to people in recovery.

- **Find your sphere of influence and work within it to advocate for recovery support services.** For example, if you work in the construction industry—where rates of substance use disorder are high—find out what your employer has to offer for people in or seeking recovery and offer to enhance whatever is already in place. Make sure your employer knows about recovery support services in your area. If you receive health insurance coverage through your employer, ask if and how much treatment is covered. If coverage is minimal, talk to your colleagues, supervisor, and others about changing coverage.

- **When election time rolls around, host house meetings for recovery-friendly candidates. Work with recovery advocates in your state to educate candidates, develop relationships with legislators, and talk to them about the importance of recovery support services where you live.**

- **If there's an interest in the recovery community where you live in starting a recovery community center, be part of grassroots organizing** by speaking out in support, talking with local leaders like city councilors, business leaders, and health care providers to find a champion, and helping to raise funds and find a suitable location.

- **Show up** at events like legislative days and recovery rallies as an important way to be a visible ally supporting people in your community.

- "Not In My Back Yard" attitudes (NIMBYism) toward recovery residences create barriers to recovery support services in many towns and cities. You can advocate for recovery housing by publicly opposing these attitudes through **letters to the editor, phone calls to city councilors, speaking at public meetings, and educating friends and neighbors** about recovery housing.

- Integrating primary care with specialty treatment (including mental health counseling and recovery support services) is an essential step toward removing barriers to recovery. Integrating these services means patients can access counseling and recovery support at the same place as primary care. Health care providers can advocate with local health care systems for this integration, and community members can look for opportunities to **serve on patient advisory groups** to educate health system administrators and health care leaders about recovery and advocate for integration.

- Syringe services programs (SSPs) are sparsely scattered across the United States, and most are underfunded. Health care providers and community members can reach out to local health care and public health organizations to advocate for starting an SSP. They can join state and federal initiatives to advocate for full funding. They can also **educate fellow community members** and speak out in favor of harm reduction in public settings.

ACRONYMS USED IN THIS BOOK

AA Alcoholics Anonymous

ACEs adverse childhood experiences

ASAM American Society of Addiction Medicine

CRP Collegiate Recovery Program

DSM-5 Diagnostic and Statistical Manual of Mental Disorders, 5th edition

FAVOR Faces and Voices of Recovery

FDA Food and Drug Administration

LGBTQ+ lesbian, gay, bisexual, trans, queer, intersex, asexual, and others

NARR National Alliance for Recovery Residences

NIDA National Institute on Drug Abuse

PCP primary care provider

PRSS peer recovery support services

RCC recovery community center

RCO recovery community organization

SAMHSA Substance Abuse and Mental Health Services Administration

SMART Self-Management and Recovery Training

SSP syringe services program

SUD substance use disorder

NOTES

Chapter 1

1 Carlyn Hood et al., "County Health Rankings: Relationships between Determinant Factors and Health Outcomes," *American Journal of Preventive Medicine* 50, no. 2 (2016): 129–135, www.doi.org/10.1016/j.amepre.2015.08.024.

2 David Williams, Michelle Sternthal, and Rosalind Wright, "Social Determinants: Taking the Social Context of Asthma Seriously," *Pediatrics* 123, Supplement 3 (2009): S174–S175.

3 Here, I expand on the ecosystem model described in Robert Ashford, Austin Brown, Rachel Ryding, and Brenda Curtis, "Building Recovery Ready Communities: The Recovery Ready Ecosystem Model and Community Framework," *Addiction Research & Theory* 28, no. 1 (2020): 1–11. The recovery ecosystem model is closely tied to William White's notion of "community recovery" and the ecology of recovery. See, for example, Arthur Evans, Roland Lamb, and William White, "The Community as Patient: Recovery-Focused Community Mobilization in Philadelphia, 2005–2012," *Alcoholism Treatment Quarterly* 31, no. 4 (2013): 450–465; and William White, "The Ecology of Recovery Revisited," Selected Papers: William L. White, October 29, 2020, www.williamwhitepapers.com/blog/2020/10/the-ecology-of-recovery-revisited.html.

4 Institute of Medicine, Committee for the Study of the Future of Public Health, "Summary and Recommendations: Why Study Public Health," *The Future of Public Health* (Washington, DC: National Academies Press, 1988), www.ncbi.nlm.nih.gov/books/NBK218215/#ddd00011.

5 US Department of Health and Human Services (HHS), Office of the Surgeon General, *Facing Addiction in America: The Surgeon General's Report on Alcohol, Drugs, and Health* (Washington, DC: HHS, November 2016), 1-4, www.addiction.surgeongeneral.gov/.

6 See, for example, comments of Gil Kerlikowske, the director of the Office of
   National Drug Control Policy under President Obama, reported in "Drug Control
   Policy Director: We Can't Arrest Our Way Out of the Drug Problem," Partnership
   to End Addiction, September 2011, https://drugfree.org/drug-and-alcohol-news
   /drug-control-policy-director-we-cant-arrest-our-way-out-of-the-drug-problem/.

7 See, for example, Jay Butler and Michael Fraser, eds., *A Public Health Guide to
   Ending the Opioid Epidemic* (New York: Oxford University Press, 2019).

8 Michelle Nolan, Bennett Allen, and Denise Paone, "Commentary on Hoots et al.
   (2019): The Gap between Evidence and Policy Calls into Question the Extent of
   a Public Health Approach to the Opioid Overdose Epidemic," *Addiction* 115, no. 5
   (2020): 959–960.

9 Hawre Jalal et al., "Changing Dynamics of the Drug Overdose Epidemic in the
   United States from 1979 through 2016," *Science* 361, no. 6408 (2018): e1184.

10 Sally Satel, "The Myth of What's Driving the Opioid Crisis," *Politico,* February 21,
   2018, www.politico.com/magazine/story/2018/02/21/the-myth-of-the-roots-of
   -the-opioid-crisis-217034/.

11 Aaron White et al., "Using Death Certificates to Explore Changes in Alcohol-
   Related Mortality in the United States, 1999 to 2017," *Alcoholism: Clinical and
   Experimental Research* 44, no. 1 (2020): 178–187.

12 This is often called the "set" and "setting" hypothesis. The "set" is the personality,
   preparation, expectations, and intention of the person using the substance, and
   "setting" is the physical, social, and cultural environment where use occurs. Ido
   Hartogsohn, "Constructing Drug Effects: A History of Set and Setting," *Drug Science, Policy and Law* 3 (2017), www.doi.org/10.1177/2050324516683325.

13 On the root causes of the opioid crisis, see, for example, Nabarun Dasgupta, Leo
   Beletsky, and Daniel Ciccarone, "Opioid Crisis: No Easy Fix to Its Social and Economic Determinants," *American Journal of Public Health* 108, no. 2 (2018): 182–186.

14 William White, "Recovery: The Next Frontier," *Counselor* 5, no. 1 (2004): 18–21.

15 Vivek Murthy, *Together: The Healing Power of Human Connection in a Sometimes
   Lonely World* (New York: HarperCollins, 2020).

16 Johann Hari, *Chasing the Scream: The First and Last Days of the War on Drugs* (New
   York: Bloomsbury, 2015), 293.

Chapter 2

1 For a thorough discussion of addiction terminology, see John Kelly, "Toward an
   Addictionary: A Proposal for More Precise Terminology," *Alcoholism Treatment
   Quarterly* 22, no. 2 (2004): 79–87, www.recoveryanswers.org/addiction-ary/.

2 American Psychiatric Association, *Diagnostic and Statistical Manual of Mental
   Disorders,* 5th ed. *(DSM-5)* (Arlington, VA: American Psychiatric Publishing, 2013).

3 Five of the *DSM-5* criteria commonly occur in individuals with severe substance use disorder (addiction): efforts to control/cut down but unable to, craving with compulsion to use, failure to fulfill roles and obligations, activities given up or reduced, and experiencing withdrawal symptoms. See Brian Coon, "The Big Five Substance Use Disorder Criteria," *Recovery Review,* October 21, 2019, www .recoveryreview.blog/2019/10/21/the-big-5-substance-use-disorder-criteria/.

4 William White has written extensively on addiction and recovery, and my writing is influenced by his work. See, for example, William White, "Addiction Recovery: Its Definition and Conceptual Boundaries," *Journal of Substance Abuse Treatment* 33, no. 3 (2007): 229–241.

5 John Kelly et al., "Prevalence and Pathways of Recovery from Drug and Alcohol Problems in the United States Population: Implications for Practice, Research, and Policy," *Drug and Alcohol Dependence* 181 (2017): 162–169.

6 HHS, *Facing Addiction in America,* 1-7.

7 Using neuroscience, Marc Lewis arrives at a different conclusion. He doesn't see addiction as a disease but rather as the result of a natural learning process that has gone too fast and too far, resulting in habits that are hard to break or "unlearn." See Marc Lewis, *The Biology of Desire: Why Addiction Is Not a Disease* (New York: PublicAffairs, 2015). Maia Szalavitz has a similar view and considers addiction a learning disability. See Maia Szalavitz, *Unbroken Brain: A Revolutionary New Way of Understanding Addiction* (New York: St. Martin's Press, 2016).

8 Recovery Research Institute, "The Brain in Recovery: The Neuroscience of Addiction Recovery," n.d., www.recoveryanswers.org/recovery-101/brain -in-recovery/.

9 National Institute on Drug Abuse, "The Science of Drug Use and Addiction: The Basics," 2018, www.drugabuse.gov/publications/media-guide/science -drug-use-addiction-basics.

10 Arthur Evans, Roland Lamb, and William White, "Promoting Intergenerational Resilience and Recovery: Policy, Clinical, and Recovery Support Strategies to Alter the Intergenerational Transmission of Alcohol, Drug, and Related Problems" (Philadelphia: Department of Behavioral Health and Intellectual disAbility Services, 2014).

11 Jeesun Jung et al., "Adverse Childhood Experiences Are Associated with High-Intensity Binge Drinking Behavior in Adulthood and Mediated by Psychiatric Disorders," *Alcohol and Alcoholism* 55, no. 2 (2020): 204–214.

12 Veterans returning from Vietnam offer solid evidence that environment influences drug use. In the early 1970s, about 10–15 percent of soldiers returning home were addicted to heroin. Between eight and twelve months later, only about 1 percent were addicted. They reported using heroin and other drugs in

Vietnam for its euphoric effects, as well as to reduce boredom, fears, and homesickness. These reasons disappeared when they returned home. Interestingly, the same research showed that soldiers who drank alcohol before serving in the war decreased their drinking while in Vietnam, and then picked it up again when they returned home. See Elisardo Becoña, "Brain Disease or Biopsychosocial Model in Addiction? Remembering the Vietnam Veteran Study," *Psicothema* 30, no. 3 (2018): 270–275.

13 Nora Volkow, Beth Han, Emily B. Einstein, and Wilson M. Compton, "Prevalence of Substance Use Disorders by Time since First Substance Use among Young People in the US," *JAMA Pediatrics* 175, no. 6 (2021): 640–643.

14 American Society of Addiction Medicine, "Definition of Addiction," 2019, www. asam.org/Quality-Science/definition-of-addiction.

15 David Courtwright, "The NIDA Brain Disease Paradigm: History, Resistance and Spinoffs," *BioSocieties* 5, no. 1 (2010): 137–147.

16 Bruce Alexander, *The Globalization of Addiction: A Study in Poverty of the Spirit* (New York: Oxford University Press, 2010).

17 Gabor Maté, *In the Realm of Hungry Ghosts* (Berkeley, CA: North Atlantic Books, 2010).

18 Hari, *Chasing the Scream.*

19 Carl Hart, *High Price* (New York: HarperCollins, 2013).

20 Brave Heart, Maria Yellow Horse, and Lemyra M. DeBruyn, "The American Indian Holocaust: Healing Historical Unresolved Grief," *American Indian and Alaska Native Mental Health Research* 8, no. 2 (1998): 56–78; and Don Coyhis, *Understanding Native American Culture: Insights for Recovery Professionals* (Colorado Springs, CO: Coyhis, 1999).

21 Hans Madueme, "Addiction and Sin: Recovery and Redemption," *AMA Journal of Ethics* 10, no. 1 (2008): 55–58.

22 Helena Hansen, *Addicted to Christ: Remaking Men in Puerto Rican Pentecostal Drug Ministries* (Oakland, CA: University of California Press, 2018).

Chapter 3

1 Recovery researcher William White suggests that the term "recovery" is "best reserved for those persons who have resolved or are in the process of resolving severe alcohol or drug related problems that meet *Diagnostic and Statistical Manual of Mental Disorders,* 4th ed. *(DSM-IV)* criteria for 'abuse' or 'dependence' [the term used at the time for the most severe form of substance use disorder]. The less medicalized terms *quit* and *cessation* more aptly describe the problem-solving processes in cases marked by less severity. The broader term *resolution* embraces both patterns of problem solving." See White, "Addiction Recovery: Its Definition and Conceptual Boundaries," 4.

2 At the same time, the media's narrative of nonwhite people in urban areas using heroin in squalid conditions didn't change. See Julie Netherland and Helena B. Hansen, "The War on Drugs That Wasn't: Wasted Whiteness, 'Dirty Doctors,' and Race in Media Coverage of Prescription Opioid Misuse," *Culture, Medicine, and Psychiatry* 40, no. 4 (2016): 664–686.

3 William White, "Waiting for Breaking Good: The Media and Addiction Recovery," Selected Papers: William L. White, March 4, 2014, www.williamwhitepapers .com/blog/2014/03/waiting-for-breaking-good-the-media-and-addiction-recovery .html.

4 William White writes that "addiction does not discriminate" as a way of saying, "'See ... it could happen to anyone ... and now you should care.' This narrative sought to normalize (aka whiten) addiction by projecting the image of 'innocent,' (aka white), middle-class children and their parents deserving of public resources to support their care. Such care was advocated as an alternative to arrest and incarceration for the 'deserving' (aka white people of means), while addiction in communities of color continued to be stigmatized, de-medicalized, and criminalized." See William White, Bill Stauffer, and Danielle Tarino, "Pillars of Stigma and Recovery Storytelling," Selected Papers: William L. White, December 3, 2020, www.williamwhitepapers.com/blog/2020/12/pillars -of-stigma-and-recovery-storytelling-bill-white-bill-stauffer-and-danielle -tarino.html.

5 Populations with low incomes are hardest hit by substance use disorder. Karin Martinson, Doug McDonald, Amy Berninger, and Kyla Wasserman, "Building Evidence-Based Strategies to Improve Employment Outcomes for Individuals with Substance Use Disorders," OPRE Report 2020-171 (Washington, DC: Office of Planning, Research, and Evaluation, Administration for Children and Families, US Department of Health and Human Services, 2021), www.acf.hhs .gov/opre/report/building-evidence-based-strategies-improve-employment -outcomes-individuals-substance.

6 Michelle Alexander, *The New Jim Crow: Mass Incarceration in the Age of Colorblindness,* 10th anniversary ed. (New York: New Press, 2020).

Chapter 4

1 Steve Sussman et al., "Spirituality in Addictions Treatment: Wisdom to Know ... What It Is," *Substance Use & Misuse* 48, no. 12 (2013): 1203.

2 In September 2006, the Betty Ford Institute convened a panel of policy makers, treatment providers, and people in recovery to develop a consensus definition of recovery, with the resulting definition: *"Recovery from substance dependence is a voluntarily maintained lifestyle characterized by sobriety, personal health, and citizenship."*

See The Betty Ford Institute Consensus Panel, "What Is Recovery? A Working Definition from the Betty Ford Institute," *Journal of Substance Abuse Treatment* 33, no. 3 (2007): 221–228. William White's definition is: *"Recovery is the experience (a process and a sustained status) through which individuals, families, and communities impacted by severe alcohol and other drug problems utilize internal and external resources to voluntarily resolve these problems, actively manage their continued vulnerability to such problems, and develop a healthy, productive, and meaningful life."* See White, "Addiction Recovery: Its Definition and Conceptual Boundaries," 229–241. In 2019, the Center for Young Adult Addiction and Recovery at Kennesaw State University in Georgia convened the Recovery Science Research Collaborative (RSRC). The group arrived at this definition: *"Recovery is an individualized, intentional, dynamic, and relational process involving sustained efforts to improve wellness."* See Robert Ashford et al., "Defining and Operationalizing the Phenomena of Recovery: A Working Definition from the Recovery Science Research Collaborative," *Addiction Research & Theory* 27, no. 3 (2019): 179–188. Additional definitions are summarized in Katie Witkiewitz, Kevin Montes, Frank Schwebel, and Jalie Tucker, "What Is Recovery?" *Alcohol Research: Current Reviews* 40, no. 3 (2020).

3 Center for Substance Abuse Treatment, *National Summit on Recovery: Conference Report* (Rockville, MD: Substance Abuse and Mental Health Services Administration, 2006); and "SAMHSA's Working Definition of Recovery," February 2012, DHHS Publication PEP12-RECDEF, www.store.samhsa.gov/sites/default/files/d7/priv/pep12-recdef.pdf.

4 Alexandre Laudet, *Environmental Scan of Measures of Recovery* (Rockville, MD: Substance Abuse and Mental Health Services Administration, 2009).

5 The US Surgeon General found that about 9.8 percent of the United States' adult population is now in remission from substance use disorder. See HHS, *Facing Addiction in America,* 5-2. In 2017, the National Recovery Survey found that 9.1 percent of the adult population "used to have a problem with drugs or alcohol but no longer do." See Kelly et al., "Prevalence and Pathways," 164. William White's review of 415 scientific reports between 1868 and 2011 found that 5.3–15.3 percent of US adults are in remission from substance use disorder. See William White, "Recovery/Remission from Substance Use Disorders: An Analysis of Reported Outcomes in 415 Scientific Reports, 1868–2011," Philadelphia Department of Behavioral Health and Intellectual DisAbility Services (2012): 2.

6 Faces and Voices of Recovery: https://facesandvoicesofrecovery.org.

7 Kelly et al., "Prevalence and Pathways," 164.

8 James Prochaska, Carlo DiClemente, and John Norcross, "In Search of How People Change: Applications to Addictive Behaviors," *American Psychologist* 47, no. 9 (1992): 1102–1114.

9   Recovery Research Institute, "Stages of Change, Stages of Recovery," www
    .recoveryanswers.org/resource/stages-of-recovery/. The graphic is based on the
    foundational work on stages of change and addiction. See Prochaska, DiClem-
    ente, and Norcross, "In Search of How People Change," 1102–1114.

10 See, for example, Terence Gorski, "Recovery: A Developmental Model," *Addiction
    and Recovery* 11, no. 2 (1991): 10–15; William White, "Stages of Recovery Model,"
    Recovery Research Institute, www.recoveryanswers.org/media
    /stages-recovery-model-william-l-white/.

11 John Kelly, Claire Greene, and Brandon Bergman, "Beyond Abstinence: Changes
    in Indices of Quality of Life with Time in Recovery in a Nationally Representa-
    tive Sample of US Adults," *Alcoholism: Clinical and Experimental Research* 42, no. 4
    (2018): 770–780.

12 David Best and Stephanie de Alwis, "Community Recovery as a Public Health
    Intervention: The Contagion of Hope," *Alcoholism Treatment Quarterly* 35, no. 3
    (2017): 187–199. See also David Best and Jo-Hanna Ivers, "Ink Spots and Ice Cream
    Cones: A Model of Recovery Contagion and Growth," *Addiction Research &
    Theory* (2021): 1–7.

13 The 2012 Life in Recovery survey identified a significant gap in our understand-
    ing about who is in recovery. Alexandre Laudet, the author of the survey report,
    stated, "At this writing, we regrettably lack the empirical knowledge base to char-
    acterize people in recovery in the United States, so we cannot definitively assess
    the representativeness of our sample relative to the recovery community at large."
    See Alexandre Laudet, "Life in Recovery: Report on the Survey Findings," Faces
    and Voices of Recovery, 2013, www.facesandvoicesofrecovery.org/wp-content/
    uploads/2019/06/22Life-in-Recovery22-Report-on-the-Survey-Findings.pdf.

14 See, for example, Alexandre Laudet and William L. White, "Recovery Capital as
    Prospective Predictor of Sustained Recovery, Life Satisfaction, and Stress among
    Former Poly-Substance Users," *Substance Use & Misuse* 43, no. 1 (2008): 27–54.

15 John Kelly, personal communication, December 10, 2020. See also John Kelly et
    al., "One-Stop Shopping for Recovery: An Investigation of Participant Character-
    istics and Benefits Derived from US Recovery Community Centers," *Alcoholism:
    Clinical and Experimental Research* 44, no. 3 (2020): 711–721.

16 HHS, *Facing Addiction in America,* 5-17.

Chapter 5

1   Young People in Recovery (YPR), a national advocacy organization founded in
    2010 by young people in recovery who wanted to help others, developed a similar
    term, "recovery-ready communities": https://youngpeopleinrecovery
    .org/advocacy/.

2 David Best, presentation at the National Alliance for Recovery Residences, Richmond, VA, October 25, 2021.

3 Laudet and White, "Recovery Capital as Prospective Predictor," 9.

4 Robert Granfield and William Cloud introduced the concept of recovery capital in 1999 as "the sum of one's total resources that can be brought to bear in an effort to overcome alcohol and drug dependence. See Robert Granfield and William Cloud, *Coming Clean: Overcoming Addiction without Treatment* (New York: NYU Press, 1999).

5 Aliza Wingo, Kerry Ressler, and Bekh Bradley, "Resilience Characteristics Mitigate Tendency for Harmful Alcohol and Illicit Drug Use in Adults with a History of Childhood Abuse: A Cross-sectional Study of 2024 Inner-City Men and Women," *Journal of Psychiatric Research* 51 (2014): 93–99.

6 William L. White, "Recovery Capital Scale," 2009, posted at www.william whitepapers.com/recovery_toolkit. Other recovery capital assessment tools include the evidence-based REC-CAP Assessment and Recovery Planning Tool developed by David Best. See the Advanced Recovery Management System website: www.recoveryoutcomes.com/rec-cap/.

7 Emily Hennessy, "Recovery Capital: A Systematic Review of the Literature," *Addiction Research & Theory* 25, no. 5 (2017): 349–360.

8 See, for example, Johanna Hanley, *The Color of Law: A Forgotten History of How Our Government Segregated America* (New York: Liveright, 2017); and Alexander, *The New Jim Crow.*

9 Researchers are also looking at what levels of support—like recovery housing—are best suited for people with different levels and types of recovery capital and levels of problem severity. For example, it may be that a person with a lot of recovery capital and a severe problem may benefit from detox followed by intense community support, whereas a person with little recovery capital and a less severe problem may benefit from residential treatment. William White and William Cloud, "Recovery Capital: A Primer for Addictions Professionals," *Counselor* 9, no. 5 (2008): 22–27.

10 David Best also calls it "reciprocal community development" and offers examples of community programs designed around this concept. See David Best, *Pathways to Recovery and Desistance* (Chicago: Policy Press, 2019).

11 David Best and Alexandre Laudet, "The Potential of Recovery Capital," RSA Peterborough Recovery Capital Project (London: RSA, 2010).

12 William White, "Recovery Is Contagious," keynote address at the Northeast Treatment (NET) Center's Consumer Council Recognition Dinner celebrating the recovery progress and service activities of NET members and the 40th anniversary of NET, April 14, 2010, Philadelphia, PA.

13 Public health professionals will recognize this as the socio-ecological model. See Kenneth McLeroy, Daniel Bibeau, Allan Steckler, and Karen Glanz, "An Ecological Perspective on Health Promotion Programs," *Health Education Quarterly* 15, no. 4 (1988): 351–377.

14 David Best, presentation at the National Alliance for Recovery Residences, Richmond, VA, October 25, 2021.

15 HHS, *Facing Addiction in America,* 5-6.

16 This book doesn't include a discussion of recovery-oriented systems of care (ROSC), which, by definition, require a systems-level change and service integration for people in recovery. That level of change is beyond the scope of work that community members can do. See, for example, Cori Sheedy and Melanie Whitter, "Guiding Principles and Elements of Recovery-Oriented Systems of Care: What Do We Know from the Research?" *Journal of Drug Addiction, Education, and Eradication* 9, no. 4 (2013): 225.

Chapter 6

1 Paraphrased from Don Coyhis and Richard Simonelli, "The Native American Healing Experience," *Substance Use & Misuse* 43, no. 12–13 (2008): 1927–1949.

2 Evans, Lamb, and White, "The Community as Patient," 450–465.

3 Research on community-based interventions is extensive. For a review article, see, for example, Kenneth McLeroy et al., "Community-Based Interventions," *American Journal of Public Health* 93, no. 4 (2003): 529–533.

4 Associated Press, *The Associated Press Stylebook,* 55th ed. (New York: Basic Books, 2020).

5 National Institute on Drug Abuse, "Principles of Adolescent Substance Use Disorder Treatment: A Research-Based Guide," January 2014, www .drugabuse.gov/publications/principles-adolescent-substance-use-disorder -treatment-research-based-guide/introduction.

6 Ken Winters and Amelia Arria, "Adolescent Brain Development and Drugs," *Prevention Researcher* 18, no. 2 (2011): 21.

7 Quoted in Kate O'Brien, "Behavior Change Case Study: Greater Portland (Maine) Council of Governments and Opioid Misuse," *Behavior Change Tactics for Urban Challenges: Insights from Practitioners,* Meeting of the Minds, February 20, 2020, https://meetingoftheminds.org/behavior-change-case-study-greater-portland -maine-council-of-governments-and-opioid-misuse-30725.

Chapter 7

1 William White describes these combinations as "patchworks, mandalas, and mosaics." William White, "Recovery Pathways Are Not Always a Pathway," Selected

Papers: William L. White, June 3, 2016, www.williamwhitepapers.com/blog /2016/06/recovery-pathways-are-not-always-a-pathway.html.

2 See Kelly et al., "Prevalence and Pathways."

3 Granfield and Cloud, *Coming Clean,* 14.

4 Robert Granfield and William Cloud, "The Elephant That No One Sees: Natural Recovery among Middle-Class Addicts," *Journal of Drug Issues* 26, no. 1 (1996): 45–61.

5 John F. Kelly, Keith Humphreys, and Marica Ferri, "Alcoholics Anonymous and Other 12-Step Programs for Alcohol Use Disorder," *Cochrane Database of Systematic Reviews* 3 (2020): 10.1002/14651858.CD012880.

6 William L. White, *Slaying the Dragon: The History of Addiction Treatment and Recovery in America* (Bloomington, IL: Chestnut Health Systems/Lighthouse Institute, 1998).

7 See, for example, Tamara Bettham et al., "Admission Practices and Cost of Care for Opioid Use Disorder at Residential Addiction Treatment Programs in the US," *Health Affairs* 40, no. 2 (February 2020).

8 Thomas Coderre, acting director of the Substance Abuse and Mental Health Services Administration, personal communication, April 6, 2020.

9 See Daniel Anderson, John McGovern, and Robert DuPont, "The Origins of the Minnesota Model of Addiction Treatment—A First Person Account," *Journal of Addictive Diseases* 18, no. 1 (1999): 107–114.

10 National Institute on Drug Abuse, *Principles of Drug Addiction Treatment: A Research-Based Guide,* 3rd ed., revised 2018, www.drugabuse.gov/publications /principles-drug-addiction-treatment-research-based-guide-third-edition/.

11 See Anne Fletcher, *Inside Rehab: The Surprising Truth about Addiction Treatment— and How to Get Help That Works* (New York: Penguin, 2013); and Lance Dodes and Zachary Dodes, *The Sober Truth: Debunking the Bad Science behind 12-Step Programs and the Rehab Industry* (Boston: Beacon Press, 2014).

12 The National Recovery Survey showed that Black people and Hispanic people are far more likely to turn to religion in recovery while at the same time not always calling their healing process "recovery." White people are less likely to turn to spirituality or religion, but they generally practice spirituality without any particular religious faith when they do. See Kelly et al., "Prevalence and Pathways."

13 Surbhi Khanna and Jeffrey M. Greeson, "A Narrative Review of Yoga and Mindfulness as Complementary Therapies for Addiction," *Complementary Therapies in Medicine* 21, no. 3 (2013): 244–252.

14 Substance Abuse and Mental Health Services Administration, *Key Substance Use and Mental Health Indicators in the United States: Results from the 2018 National Survey on Drug Use and Health,* HHS Publication No. PEP19-5068, NSDUH Series H-54

(Rockville, MD: Center for Behavioral Health Statistics and Quality, Substance Abuse and Mental Health Services Administration, 2019). See table 1.4, p. A-5.

15 White, "Recovery/Remission," 2.

16 John Kelly et al., "How Many Recovery Attempts Does It Take to Successfully Resolve an Alcohol or Drug Problem? Estimates and Correlates from a National Study of Recovering US Adults," *Alcoholism: Clinical and Experimental Research* 43, no. 7 (2019): 1533–1544. For number of quit attempts for cigarette smoking, see Michael Chaiton et al., "Estimating the Number of Quit Attempts It Takes to Quit Smoking Successfully in a Longitudinal Cohort of Smokers," *BMJ Open* 6, no. 6 (2016).

Chapter 8

1 In keeping with AA's tradition of anonymity, the names of the people I interviewed for this chapter are not their real names.

2 The discussion of Alcoholics Anonymous in this chapter draws from White, *Slaying the Dragon,* 169–211.

3 Alcoholics Anonymous, *Twelve Steps and Twelve Traditions* (New York: Alcoholics Anonymous World Services, 1981).

4 Kelly et al., "Prevalence and Pathways."

5 The Cochrane Collaboration reviewed randomized controlled trials, the highest standard for scientific inquiry in the health care field. See Kelly, Humphreys, and Ferri, "Alcoholics Anonymous and Other 12-Step Programs."

6 William White, Marc Galenter, Keith Humphreys, and John Kelly, "We Do Recover: Scientific Studies on Narcotics Anonymous," unpublished paper, April 10, 2020, www.williamwhitepapers.com/blog/2020/04/we-do-recover -scientific-studies-of-na.html.

7 Laura Monico et al., "Buprenorphine Treatment and 12-Step Meeting Attendance: Conflicts, Compatibilities, and Patient Outcomes," *Journal of Substance Abuse Treatment* 57 (2015): 89–95.

8 John Kelly, Molly Magill, and Robert Lauren Stout, "How Do People Recover from Alcohol Dependence? A Systematic Review of the Research on Mechanisms of Behavior Change in Alcoholics Anonymous," *Addiction Research & Theory* 17, no. 3 (2009): 236–259.

9 Frank Martela, "Helping Others Is Good for Your Health: Research Confirms the Positive Health Impact of Being Good to Others," *Psychology Today,* September 4, 2020, www.psychologytoday.com/us/blog/insights-more -meaningful-existence/202009/helping-others-is-good-your-health.

10 Kelly, Magill, and Stout, "How Do People Recover from Alcohol Dependence?" 249.

Chapter 9

1 Lawrence Yang, Liang Wong, Margaux Grivel, and Deborah Hasin, "Stigma and Substance Use Disorders: An International Phenomenon," *Current Opinion in Psychiatry* 30, no. 5 (2017): 378.

2 Centers for Disease Control and Prevention, "Opioid Overdose: Understanding the Epidemic," March 17, 2021, www.cdc.gov/opioids/basics/epidemic.html.

3 Utsha Khatri et al., "Racial/Ethnic Disparities in Unintentional Fatal and Nonfatal Emergency Medical Services–Attended Opioid Overdoses during the COVID-19 Pandemic in Philadelphia," *JAMA Network Open* 4, no. 1 (2021): e2034878.

4 Jasmine Drake et al., "Exploring the Impact of the Opioid Epidemic in Black and Hispanic Communities in the United States," *Drug Science, Policy and Law* 6 (2020): 2050324520940428.

5 Lloyd Johnston et al., "Monitoring the Future National Survey Results on Drug Use, 1975–2020: Overview, Key Findings on Adolescent Drug Use," *Institute for Social Research* 2021: p. 35 (marijuana) and p. 38 (alcohol).

6 White, Stauffer, and Tarino, "Pillars of Stigma and Recovery Storytelling."

7 National Academies of Sciences, Engineering, and Medicine, *Ending Discrimination against People with Mental and Substance Use Disorders: The Evidence for Stigma Change* (Washington, DC: National Academies of Sciences, Engineering, and Medicine, 2016), www.ncbi.nlm.nih.gov/books/NBK384923/. Most of chapter 9 relies on the research cited in this report.

8 William White, "Long-Term Strategies to Reduce the Stigma Attached to Addiction, Treatment, and Recovery within the City of Philadelphia (with Particular Reference to Medication-Assisted Treatment/Recovery)," Philadelphia: Department of Behavioral Health and Mental Retardation Services (2009).

9 Even after a court settlement in 2018 with a Massachusetts nursing facility for violating anti-discrimination laws for rejecting people with opioid use disorder, discrimination continued. Simeone Kimmel et al., "Rejection of Patients with Opioid Use Disorder Referred for Post-acute Medical Care before and after an Anti-discrimination Settlement in Massachusetts," *Journal of Addiction Medicine* 15, no. 1 (2021): 20–26.

10 Dr. Alane O'Connor, addiction medicine specialist and clinical advisor, Maine Maternal Opioid Misuse Initiative, personal communication, August 22, 2021.

11 Even "substance abuse," the old medical term for substance use disorder and still widely used, carries negative connotations that can affect the way patients see themselves. See Kelly, "Toward an Addictionary," 79–87.

12 See Katherine Keyes et al., "Stigma and Treatment for Alcohol Disorders in the United States," *American Journal of Epidemiology* 172, no. 12 (2010): 1364–1372; and Loren Brener et al., "Perceptions of Discriminatory Treatment by Staff as

Predictors of Drug Treatment Completion: Utility of a Mixed Methods Approach," *Drug and Alcohol Review* 29, no. 5 (2010): 491–497.

13 Research shows that people think a "substance abuser" is personally responsible for their condition and in need of punishment, compared with a "person with substance use disorder," who is sick and in need of treatment. See John Kelly and Cassandra M. Westerhoff, "Does It Matter How We Refer to Individuals with Substance-Related Conditions? A Randomized Study of Two Commonly Used Terms," *International Journal of Drug Policy* 21, no. 3 (2010): 202–207.

14 National Institute on Drug Abuse, "Words Matter: Preferred Language for Talking about Addiction: Terms to Use and Avoid When Talking about Addiction," June 21, 2021, www.drugabuse.gov/drug-topics/addiction-science/words-matter-preferred -language-talking-about-addiction#table.

15 Maia Szalavitz, "Why We Should De-criminalize All Drugs," *The Guardian*, November 18, 2016, www.theguardian.com/us-news/commentisfree/2016/jul/05 /why-de-criminalize-all-drugs-stigma.

16 Research on reducing stigma related to substance use disorders follows earlier research on reducing the stigma associated with mental health conditions. See, for example, Patrick Corrigan et al., "Challenging the Public Stigma of Mental Illness: A Meta-analysis of Outcome Studies," *Psychiatric Services* 63, no. 10 (2012): 963–973; James Livingston, Teresa Milne, Mei Lan Fang, and Erica Amari, "The Effectiveness of Interventions for Reducing Stigma Related to Substance Use Disorders: A Systematic Review," *Addiction* 107, no. 1 (2012): 39–50; and Nisha Mehta et al., "Evidence for Effective Interventions to Reduce Mental Health– Related Stigma and Discrimination in the Medium and Long Term: Systematic Review," *British Journal of Psychiatry* 207, no. 5 (2015): 377–384.

17 Professionals view the "substance abuser" as less likely to benefit from treat-ment and more likely to benefit from punishment, more likely to be threatening and blamed for their substance use problems, and more able to control their substance use without help, compared with the "person with substance use dis-order." See John Kelly, Sarah Dow, and Cara Westerhoff, "Does Our Choice of Substance-Related Terms Influence Perceptions of Treatment Need? An Empiri-cal Investigation with Two Commonly Used Terms," *Journal of Drug Issues* 40, no. 4 (2010): 805–818.

18 Mental health professionals thought that "substance abusers" were personally responsible for their actions and should receive punishment instead of therapy. See Kelly and Westerhoff, "Does It Matter How We Refer to Individuals with Substance-Related Conditions?"

19 Nurses are more judgmental than other health care professionals toward patients who misuse drugs. See Matthew Howard and Sulki Chung, "Nurses' Attitudes

toward Substance Misusers. II. Experiments and Studies Comparing Nurses to Other Groups," *Substance Use & Misuse* 35, no. 4 (2000): 503–532.

20 Diana Clarke et al., "Emergency Department Staff Attitudes towards Mental Health Consumers: A Literature Review and Thematic Content Analysis," *International Journal of Mental Health Nursing* 23, no. 3 (2014): 273–284.

21 John Kelly, Claire Greene, and Alexandra Abry, "A US National Randomized Study to Guide How Best to Reduce Stigma When Describing Drug-Related Impairment in Practice and Policy," *Addiction* 116, no. 7 (2021): 1757–1767.

22 Emma McGinty et al., "Portraying Mental Illness and Drug Addiction as Treatable Health Conditions: Effects of a Randomized Experiment on Stigma and Discrimination," *Social Science & Medicine* 126 (2015): 73–85.

23 Emma McGinty et al., "Communication Strategies to Counter Stigma and Improve Mental Illness and Substance Use Disorder Policy," *Psychiatric Services* 69, no. 2 (2018): 136–146.

Chapter 10

1 See Network for Public Health Law, "Legal Interventions to Reduce Overdose Mortality: Naloxone Access Laws," July 1, 2020, www.networkforphl.org/resources /legal-interventions-to-reduce-overdose-mortality-naloxone-access-and-good -samaritan-laws/.

2 Drug Policy Alliance, n.d., "Syringe Access," https://drugpolicy.org/issues /syringe-access.

3 Caitlin Conrad et al., "Community Outbreak of HIV Infection Linked to Injection Drug Use of Oxymorphone—Indiana, 2015," *Morbidity and Mortality Weekly Report* 64, no. 16 (May 1, 2015): 443–444.

4 WBIW.com, "Scott County Commissioners Vote to End Syringe Services Program," June 3, 2021, www.wbiw.com/2021/06/03/scott-county-commissioners -vote-to-end-syringe-services-program/.

5 Centers for Disease Control and Prevention, "Syringe Services Programs (SSPs)," May 23, 2019, www.cdc.gov/ssp/index.html.

6 Alexander Lekhtman, "Congress Plans Historic Federal Funding for Syringe Programs," *Filter* magazine, July 22, 2021, https://filtermag.org /congress-funding-syringe-programs/.

7 Chloé Potier et al., "Supervised Injection Services: What Has Been Demonstrated? A Systematic Literature Review," *Drug and Alcohol Dependence* 145 (2014): 48–68.

8 US Department of Justice, "Appellate Court Agrees with Government That Supervised Injection Sites Are Illegal under Federal Law; Reverses District Court

Ruling," press release, January 24, 2021, www.justice.gov/opa/pr/appellate-court
-agrees-government-supervised-injection-sites-are-illegal-under-federal-law.
On New York's overdose prevention sites, see Drug Policy Alliance, "New York
City to Open Nation's First-Ever Overdose Prevention Center Pilots to Save
Lives Amid Record Overdoses," November 30, 2021, https://drugpolicy.org/press
-release/2021/11/new-york-city-open-nations-first-ever-overdose-prevention-center
-pilots-save

9 Kastalia Medrano, "For Maine's Church of Safe Injection, a Bittersweet Legalization," *Filter* magazine, October 7, 2021.https://filtermag.org/maine-church-of
-safe-injection/?fbclid=IwARogbyWPfwmOCDhquQiCuKKowkC2SePpUSy
-5HYaP8Je31_wASZMSni6LIo

10 Colleen Cowles, *War on Us: How the War on Drugs and Myths about Addiction Have
Created a War on All of Us* (St. Paul, MN: Fidalgo Press, 2019).

11 Alexander, *The New Jim Crow.*

12 Alexis Kuerbis et al., "Profiles of Confidence and Commitment to Change as
Predictors of Moderated Drinking: A Person-Centered Approach," *Psychology of
Addictive Behaviors* 28, no. 4 (2014): 1065.

13 Marlous Tuithof et al., "Alcohol Consumption and Symptoms as Predictors for
Relapse of DSM-5 Alcohol Use Disorder," *Drug and Alcohol Dependence* 140 (2014):
85–91.

Chapter 11

1 Substance Abuse and Mental Health Services Administration, *SAMHSA's Concept
of Trauma and Guidance for a Trauma-Informed Approach,* HHS Publication No.
(SMA) 14-4884 (Rockville, MD: Substance Abuse and Mental Health Services
Administration, 2014).

2 Jamie Marich, *Trauma and the 12 Steps, Revised and Expanded: An Inclusive Guide to
Enhancing Recovery* (Berkeley, CA: North Atlantic Books, 2020).

3 See, for example, *SAMHSA's Concept of Trauma and Guidance for a Trauma-
Informed Approach.*

4 Vincent Felitti et al., "Relationship of Childhood Abuse and Household Dysfunction to Many of the Leading Causes of Death in Adults: The Adverse Childhood Experiences (ACE) Study," *American Journal of Preventive Medicine* 14, no. 4
(1998): 245–258.

5 Howard Pinderhughes, Rachel Davis, and Myesha Williams, *Adverse Community
Experiences and Resilience: A Framework for Addressing and Preventing Community
Trauma* (Oakland, CA: Prevention Institute, 2015).

6 Dodes and Dodes, *The Sober Truth.*

7   Marich, *Trauma and the 12 Steps.*
8   HHS, *Facing Addiction in America,* 2-22.
9   National Institute on Drug Abuse, "The Connection between Substance Use Disorders and Mental Illness," April 13, 2021, www.drugabuse.gov/publications /research-reports/common-comorbidities-substance-use-disorders/part-1 -connection-between-substance-use-disorders-mental-illness.
10 Bessel van der Kolk, *The Body Keeps the Score: Brain, Mind, and Body in the Healing of Trauma* (New York: Penguin Books, 2015), 352.

Chapter 12

1   Thomas Coderre, personal communication, April 6, 2020.
2   Christy Scott and Michael Dennis, *Recovery Management Checkups: An Early Reintervention Model* (Chicago: Chestnut Health Systems, 2003), 6.
3   John Kelly and William White, eds., *Addiction Recovery Management: Theory, Research, and Practice* (New York: Springer Science & Business Media, 2010).
4   Centers for Disease Control and Prevention, "Smoking and Cancer," April 2, 2021, www.cdc.gov/tobacco/campaign/tips/diseases/cancer.html.
5   National Institute on Drug Abuse, "HIV, Hepatitis, and Other Infectious Diseases," June 2020, www.drugabuse.gov/drug-topics/health-consequences -drug-misuse/hiv-hepatitis-other-infectious-diseases.
6   National Institute on Drug Abuse, "Respiratory Effects," June 15, 2020, www .drugabuse.gov/drug-topics/health-consequences-drug-misuse/respiratory -effects.
7   Nearly all drugs affect the cardiovascular system. National Institute on Drug Abuse, "Cardiovascular Effects," June 15, 2020, www.drugabuse.gov/drug-topics /health-consequences-drug-misuse/cardiovascular-effects.
8   Mandy Stahre et al., "Contribution of Excessive Alcohol Consumption to Deaths and Years of Potential Life Lost in the United States," *Preventing Chronic Disease* 11 (June 26, 2014): 11: E109, www.doi.org/10.5888/pcd11.130293.
9   Some drugs, like methamphetamine, opioids, and some prescription drugs, cause "dry mouth," which promotes dental disease. Smoking cigarettes can also lead to gum disease and tooth loss. See Mohsen Yazdanian et al., "Dental Caries and Periodontal Disease among People Who Use Drugs: A Systematic Review and Meta-analysis," *BMC Oral Health* 20, no. 1 (2020): 1–18.
10 Felitti et al., "Relationship of Childhood Abuse and Household Dysfunction."
11 van der Kolk, *The Body Keeps the Score.*
12 Clinicians used to think that quitting both drugs (or alcohol) and cigarettes at the same time was too difficult and would result in bad outcomes for addiction

treatment. New research, however, shows that this isn't the case. See Andrea Weinberger, Allison Funk, and Renee Goodwin, "A Review of Epidemiologic Research on Smoking Behavior among Persons with Alcohol and Illicit Substance Use Disorders," *Preventive Medicine* 92 (2016): 148–159, p. 157.

13 US Department of Health and Human Services, *Smoking Cessation: A Report of the Surgeon General* (Atlanta, GA: US Department of Health and Human Services, Centers for Disease Control and Prevention, National Center for Chronic Disease Prevention and Health Promotion, Office on Smoking and Health, 2020), www.hhs.gov/sites/default/files/2020-cessation-sgr-full-report.pdf.

14 For example, using tobacco and alcohol together is associated with a greater risk of head and neck cancer, cirrhosis, and pancreatitis than the use of alcohol alone. See Weinberger, Funk, and Goodwin, "A Review of Epidemiologic Research," 148.

15 Benjamin Taylor and Jürgen Rehm, "When Risk Factors Combine: The Interaction between Alcohol and Smoking for Aerodigestive Cancer, Coronary Heart Disease, and Traffic and Fire Injury," *Addictive Behaviors* 31, no. 9 (2006): 1522–1535.

16 David Eddie et al., "Medical Burden of Disease among Individuals in Recovery from Alcohol and Other Drug Problems in the United States: Findings from the National Recovery Survey," *Journal of Addiction Medicine* 13, no. 5 (2019): 385–395.

17 Andrea Weinberger et al., "Cigarette Smoking Is Associated with Increased Risk of Substance Use Disorder Relapse: A Nationally Representative, Prospective Longitudinal Investigation," *Journal of Clinical Psychiatry* 78, no. 2 (2017): e152.

18 National Institute on Drug Abuse, "Comorbidity: Substance Use Disorders and Other Mental Illnesses Drug Facts," August 1, 2018, www.drugabuse.gov /publications/drugfacts/comorbidity-substance-use-disorders-other-mental -illnesses.

19 National Institute on Drug Abuse, "The Connection between Substance Use Disorders and Mental Illness."

20 Eddie et al., "Medical Burden of Disease."

21 Jane Quinlan and Felicia Cox, "Acute Pain Management in Patients with Drug Dependence Syndrome," *Pain Reports* 2, no. 4 (2017).

22 Substance Abuse and Mental Health Services Administration, *Managing Chronic Pain in Adults with or in Recovery from Substance Use Disorders,* Treatment Improvement Protocol (TIP) Series 54, HHS Publication No. (SMA) 12-4671 (Rockville, MD: Substance Abuse and Mental Health Services Administration, 2011).

23 Deborah Dowell, Tamara Haegerich, and Roger Chou, "CDC Guideline for Prescribing Opioids for Chronic Pain—United States, 2016," *MMWR Recommendations and Report* 65, no. RR-1 (2016): 1–49.

24 Nora Volkow, "Stigma and the Toll of Addiction," *New England Journal of Medicine* 382, no. 14 (2020): 1289–1290.

25 HHS, *Facing Addiction in America,* chapter 6.

26 From Robert Drake et al., "A Review of Treatments for People with Severe Mental Illnesses and Co-occurring Substance Use Disorders," *Psychiatric Rehabilitation Journal* 27, no. 4 (2004): 360, quoted in Larry Davidson and William White, "The Concept of Recovery as an Organizing Principle for Integrating Mental Health and Addiction Services," *Journal of Behavioral Health Services & Research* 34, no. 2 (2007): 109–120.

27 William White, *Recovery Management and Recovery-Oriented Systems of Care* (Chicago: Great Lakes Addiction Technology Transfer Center, Northeast Addiction Technology Transfer Center, and Philadelphia Department of Behavioral Health and Mental Retardation Services, 2008).

28 HealthCare.gov, "Health Benefits and Coverage: What Marketplace Health Insurance Plans Cover," n.d., www.healthcare.gov/coverage/what-marketplace-plans-cover/.

29 Kendall Jeynes and E. Leigh Gibson, "The Importance of Nutrition in Aiding Recovery from Substance Use Disorders: A Review," *Drug and Alcohol Dependence* 179 (2017): 229–239.

30 Mateja Savoie-Roskos et al., "Diet, Nutrition, and Substance Use Disorder," Utah State University Extension factsheet, July 21, 2020, https://digitalcommons.usu.edu/extension_curall/2121/.

31 Jorge Giménez-Meseguer, Juan Tortosa-Martínez, and Juan M. Cortell-Tormo, "The Benefits of Physical Exercise on Mental Disorders and Quality of Life in Substance Use Disorders Patients: Systematic Review and Meta-analysis," *International Journal of Environmental Research and Public Health* 17, no. 10 (2020): 3680.

32 Elisabeth Zschucke, Andreas Heinz, and Ströhle Andreas, "Exercise and Physical Activity in the Therapy of Substance Use Disorders," *Scientific World Journal* (2012): 901741, www.doi.org/10.1100/2012/901741.#xad;doi>

33 Katherine Kaplan et al., "An Evidence-Based Review of Insomnia Treatment in Early Recovery," *Journal of Addiction Medicine* 8, no. 6 (2014): 389–394.

34 Edo Shonin and William Van Gordon, "The Mechanisms of Mindfulness in the Treatment of Mental Illness and Addiction," *International Journal of Mental Health and Addiction* 14, no. 5 (2016): 844–849.

35 Surbhi Khanna and Jeffrey M. Greeson, "A Narrative Review of Yoga and Mindfulness as Complementary Therapies for Addiction," *Complementary Therapies in Medicine* 21, no. 3 (2013): 244–252.

36 White et al., "Using Death Certificates."

Chapter 13

1 Jeffrey Munn, *Staying Sober without God: The Practical 12 Steps to Long-Term Recovery from Alcoholism and Addictions* (self-published, 2019).

2 Steve Sussman et al., "Spirituality in Addictions Treatment."

3 Keith Humphreys, *Circles of Recovery: Self-Help Organizations for Addictions* (Cambridge: Cambridge University Press, 2003).

4 *Recovery Dharma: How to Use Buddhist Practices and Principles to Heal the Suffering of Addiction* (independently published by Recovery Dharma, July 30, 2019).

5 Simon Goldberg et al., "The Empirical Status of Mindfulness-Based Interventions: A Systematic Review of 44 Meta-analyses of Randomized Controlled Trials," *Perspectives on Psychological Science* (2021): 1745691620968771.

6 Feifei Wang and Attila Szabo, "Effects of Yoga on Stress among Healthy Adults: A Systematic Review," *Alternative Therapies in Health & Medicine* 26, no. 4 (2020).

7 John Kelly and David Eddie, "The Role of Spirituality and Religiousness in Aiding Recovery from Alcohol and Other Drug Problems: An Investigation in a National US Sample," *Psychology of Religion and Spirituality* 12, no. 1 (2020): 116.

8 Sussman et al., "Spirituality in Addictions Treatment."

9 J. Scott Tonigan, Kristina Rynes, and Barbara McCrady, "Spirituality as a Change Mechanism in 12-Step Programs: A Replication, Extension, and Refinement," *Substance Use & Misuse* 48, no. 12 (2013): 1161–1173.

10 Audrey Hang Hai et al., "The Efficacy of Spiritual/Religious Interventions for Substance Use Problems: A Systematic Review and Meta-analysis of Randomized Controlled Trials," *Drug and Alcohol Dependence* 202 (2019): 134–148.

11 AA's effectiveness may be through social connections, informal one-on-one coaching by sponsors, and role models in other members in the program who demonstrate how to stay sober and inspire hope by the lives they lead. See John Kelly, "Is Alcoholics Anonymous Religious, Spiritual, Neither? Findings from 25 Years of Mechanisms of Behavior Change Research," *Addiction* 112, no. 6 (2017): 929–936.

12 Kelly, Humphreys, and Ferri, "Alcoholics Anonymous and Other 12-Step Programs."

Chapter 14

1 Portions of this chapter were published earlier in Alison Jones Webb, "Medication Assistance," *Journey Magazine,* issue 11 (October 2020).

3 Boston Medical Center, "Reducing Stigma: Why Words about Addiction Matter," n.d., www.bmc.org/addiction/reducing-stigma; National Harm Reduction Coalition, "Pregnancy and Substance Use: A Harm Reduction Toolkit," September 24,

2021, https://harmreduction.org/issues/pregnancy-and-substance-use-a-harm
-reduction-toolkit/.

4   Robert Ashford, Austin Brown, and Brenda Curtis, "Substance Use, Recovery,
    and Linguistics: The Impact of Word Choice on Explicit and Implicit Bias,"
    Drug and Alcohol Dependence 189 (2018): 131–138.

5   For a comprehensive look at medications for addiction, see Substance Abuse
    and Mental Health Services Administration, *Medications for Opioid Use Disorder,*
    Treatment Improvement Protocol (TIP) Series 63, HHS Publication No. PEP20-
    02-01-006 (Rockville, MD: Substance Abuse and Mental Health Services Admin-
    istration, 2020).

6   Noa Krawczyk et al., "Opioid Agonist Treatment and Fatal Overdose Risk in a
    State-wide US Population Receiving Opioid Use Disorder Services," *Addiction* 115,
    no. 9 (2020): 1683–1694.

7   US Department of Health and Human Services, "Practice Guidelines for the
    Administration of Buprenorphine for Treating Opioid Use Disorder," *Federal
    Register* 86, no. 80 (April 28, 2021): 22439–22440.

8   The US Drug Enforcement Administration classifies substances into five catego-
    ries, based on the substance's medical use and potential for dependence/addic-
    tion. Schedule I drugs are the most likely to cause dependence, have no medical
    use, and are illegal. Schedule V drugs are the least likely to lead to dependence.
    Methadone is a Schedule II drug, and buprenorphine is a Schedule III drug. See
    the US Drug Enforcement Administration, "Drug Scheduling," n.d., www.dea
    .gov/drug-information/drug-scheduling.

9   Sarah Wakeman et al., "Effect of Integrating Substance Use Disorder Treatment
    into Primary Care on Inpatient and Emergency Department Utilization," *Journal
    of General Internal Medicine* 34, no. 6 (2019): 871–877.

10 Gail D'Onofrio et al., "Emergency Department–Initiated Buprenorphine/Nalox-
    one Treatment for Opioid Dependence: A Randomized Clinical Trial," *JAMA* 313,
    no. 16 (2015): 1636–1644.

11 Arthur Williams et al., "Acute Care, Prescription Opioid Use, and Overdose Fol-
    lowing Discontinuation of Long-Term Buprenorphine Treatment for Opioid Use
    Disorder," *American Journal of Psychiatry* 177, no. 2 (2020): 117–124.

12 Monico et al., "Buprenorphine Treatment."

13 Mary Peeler et al., "Racial and Ethnic Disparities in Maternal and Infant Out-
    comes among Opioid-Exposed-Mother-Infant-Dyads in Massachusetts (2017–2019),"
    American Journal of Public Health 110, no. 12 (2020): 1828–1836.

14 Alane O'Connor et al., "Predictors of Treatment Retention in Postpartum Women
    Prescribed Buprenorphine during Pregnancy," *Journal of Substance Abuse Treat-
    ment* 86 (2018): 26–29.

Chapter 15

1   Portions of this chapter were published earlier in Alison Jones Webb, "Recovery Residences," *Journey Magazine,* issue 10 (August 2020).

2   The term "halfway house" is used to describe several types of transitional housing, including residential facilities that are part of the carceral system for people leaving jail or prison, often on probation. The "half" refers to "half free, half imprisoned." Some residents in recovery residences may be transitioning out of incarceration, but that is not a condition for living there.

3   I am indebted to David Sheridan for information on the history of recovery residences and a discussion on the importance of recovery residences in building recovery capital.

4   Steven Melemis, "Relapse Prevention and the Five Rules of Recovery," *Yale Journal of Biology and Medicine* 88, no. 3 (2015): 325–332.

5   Sean McCabe, James Cranford, and Carol Boyd, "Stressful Events and Other Predictors of Remission from Drug Dependence in the United States: Longitudinal Results from a National Survey," *Journal of Substance Abuse Treatment* 71 (2016): 41–47.

6   The social model contrasts with the medical model of treatment and recovery, where care is for an acute situation and a person is taken away from the community and placed in residential treatment. See Douglas Polcin et al., "Maximizing Social Model Principles in Residential Recovery Settings," *Journal of Psychoactive Drugs* 46, no. 5 (2014): 436–443.

7   Substance Abuse and Mental Health Services Administration, *Recovery Housing: Best Practices and Suggested Guidelines,* 2018, www.samhsa.gov /resource/ebp/recovery-housing-best-practices-suggested-guidelines.

8   Alexandre Laudet and Keith Humphreys, "Promoting Recovery in an Evolving Policy Context: What Do We Know and What Do We Need to Know about Recovery Support Services?" *Journal of Substance Abuse Treatment* 45, no. 1 (2013): 126–133.

9   Douglas Polcin et al., "What Did We Learn from Our Study on Sober Living Houses and Where Do We Go from Here?" *Journal of Psychoactive Drugs* 42, no. 4 (2010): 425–433.

10 Anthony Lo Sasso et al., "Benefits and Costs Associated with Mutual-Help Community-Based Recovery Homes: The Oxford House Model," *Evaluation and Program Planning* 35, no. 1 (2012): 47–53.

11 Douglas Polcin et al., "Community Context of Sober Living Houses," *Addiction Research & Theory* 20, no. 6 (2012): 480–491.

12 I'm grateful to Dave Sheridan, executive director of the National Alliance for Recovery Residences, and Dr. Ronald Springel, executive director of the Maine

Association of Recovery Residences, for in-depth discussions about recovery residences as part of the continuum of care for people in recovery.

13 Amy Mericle et al., "Distribution and Neighborhood Correlates of Sober Living House Locations in Los Angeles," *American Journal of Community Psychology* 58, no. 1–2 (2016): 89–99.

14 See National Alliance for Recovery Residences, Center for Social Innovation, and the National Council for Behavioral Health, *Helping Recovery Residences Adapt to Support People with Medication-Assisted Recovery*, n.d., www .thenationalcouncil.org/topics/addictions/3-18-19narr-c4-ncbh_mar-rh-brief/.

15 Jennifer Miles et al., "Supporting Individuals Using Medications for Opioid Use Disorder in Recovery Residences: Challenges and Opportunities for Addressing the Opioid Epidemic," *American Journal of Drug and Alcohol Abuse* 46, no. 3 (2020): 266–272.

16 Ivan Cano et al., "Recovery Capital Pathways: Modelling the Components of Recovery Wellbeing," *Drug and Alcohol Dependence* 181 (2017): 11–19.

17 Polcin et al., "Community Context of Sober Living Houses."

Chapter 16

1 Laudet and Humphreys, "Promoting Recovery in an Evolving Policy Context."

2 US Department of Housing and Urban Development, "Housing Discrimination under the Fair Housing Act," n.d., www.hud.gov/program_offices /fair_housing_equal_opp/fair_housing_act_overview,

3 US Department of Housing and Urban Development, "Office of General Counsel Guidance on Application of Fair Housing Act Standards to the Use of Criminal Records by Providers of Housing and Real Estate-Related Transactions," April 4, 2016, www.hud.gov/sites/documents/hud_ogcguidappfhastandcr.pdf.

4 Susan Pfefferle, Samantha Karon, and Brandy Wyant, *Choice Matters: Housing Models That May Promote Recovery for Individuals and Families Facing Opioid Use Disorder* (Washington, DC: Office of the Assistant Secretary for Planning and Evaluation, US Department of Health and Human Services, June 23, 2019), www .aspe.hhs.gov/reports/choice-matters-housing-models-may-promote-recovery -individuals-families-facing-opioid-use-disorder-0.

Chapter 17

1 Roger Duncan, "The Why of Work: Purpose and Meaning Really Do Matter," *Forbes* magazine, September 11, 2018, www.forbes.com/sites/rodgerdeanduncan /2018/09/11/the-why-of-work-purpose-and-meaning-really-do-matter /?sh=181b30eb68e1.

2   Eric Goplerud, Sarah Hodge, and Tess Benham, "A Substance Use Cost Cal-
    culator for US Employers with an Emphasis on Prescription Pain Medication
    Misuse," *Journal of Occupational and Environmental Medicine* 59, no. 11 (2017): 1063,
    www.doi.org/10.1097/JOM.0000000000001157.

3   David Eddie et al., "From Working on Recovery to Working in Recovery:
    Employment Status among a Nationally Representative US Sample of Individu-
    als Who Have Resolved a Significant Alcohol or Other Drug Problem," *Journal of
    Substance Abuse Treatment* 113 (2020): 108000.

4   Karin Martinson et al., *Building Evidence-Based Strategies to Improve Employment
    Outcomes for Individuals with Substance Use Disorders.*

5   See Eddie et al., "From Working on Recovery to Working in Recovery."

6   ADA National Network, "The ADA, Addiction, Recovery, and Employment,"
    2020, https://adata.org/factsheet/ada-addiction-recovery-and-employment.

7   Martinson et al., *Building Evidence-Based Strategies.*

8   Gary Fields and John Emshwiller, "As Arrest Records Rise, Americans Find
    Consequences Can Last a Lifetime: Even if Charges Were Dropped, a Lingering
    Arrest Record Can Ruin Chances of a Job," *Wall Street Journal,* August 18, 2014,
    www.wsj.com/articles/as-arrest-records-rise-americans-find-consequences-can
    -last-a-lifetime-1408415402.

9   Recovery Centers of America, *Economic Cost of Substance Abuse in the United
    States, 2016,* September 2017, https://recoverycentersofamerica.com/economic
    -cost-substance-abuse/.

10 Center for Behavioral Health Statistics and Quality, *National Survey on Drug Use
    and Health: 2013 Dress Rehearsal Final Report* (Rockville, MD: Substance Abuse
    and Mental Health Services Administration, 2014).

11 Being a Recovery Friendly Workplace isn't the same as being a drug-free work-
    place, which is a program required for organizations with federally funded
    projects. See Substance Abuse and Mental Health Services Administration,
    "Drug-Free Workplace Programs," January 12, 2022, www.samhsa.gov
    /workplace.

Chapter 18

1   Parts of Andrew's story recounted here are from his online post, "Reflecting on
    My Addiction and Recovery, Then and Now," Partnership to End Addiction,
    April 2020, https://drugfree.org/parent-blog/reflecting-on-my-addiction-and-
    recovery-then-and-now/?fbclid=IwAR0fZT32zCDDpp_b6vKwrnRU4CIa
    PDQJcihKu_hD6O33WsnqIx-bsp18MPU.

2   I am indebted to Lisa Laitman, director of the Alcohol and Other Drug Assis-
    tance Program at Rutgers University, for inviting me to New Brunswick and

sharing her knowledge, wisdom, and experience in developing and running the Rutgers Collegiate Recovery Program.

3 Noel Vest et al., "College Programming for Students in Addiction Recovery: A PRISMA-Guided Scoping Review," *Addictive Behaviors* 121 (2021): 106992, p. 2.

4 Association of Recovery in Higher Education website: https:// collegiaterecovery.org/crps-crcs/.

5 Alexandre Laudet et al., "In College and In Recovery: Reasons for Joining a Collegiate Recovery Program," *Journal of American College Health* 64, no. 3 (2016): 238–246.

6 Alexandre Laudet et al., "Characteristics of Students Participating in Collegiate Recovery Programs: A National Survey," *Journal of Substance Abuse Treatment* 51 (2015): 38–46.

7 Kitty Harris et al., "Achieving Systems-Based Sustained Recovery: A Comprehensive Model for Collegiate Recovery Communities," *Journal of Groups in Addiction & Recovery* 2, no. 2–4 (2008): 220–237.

8 Alexandre Laudet et al., "Collegiate Recovery Programs: Results from the First National Survey," presented at the 4th Annual Conference on Collegiate Recovery, April 3–5, 2013, Texas Tech University, Lubbock, TX.

9 Alexandre Laudet et al., "Collegiate Recovery Communities Programs: What Do We Know and What Do We Need to Know?" *Journal of Social Work Practice in the Addictions* 14, no. 1 (2014): 84–100.

10 Emily Hennessy et al., "Protocol for a Systematic Review: Recovery Schools for Improving Well-Being among Students in Recovery from Substance Use Disorders: A Systematic Review," *Campbell Systematic Reviews* 13, no. 1 (2017): 1–39.

11 Association of Recovery Schools website: https://recoveryschools.org/find -a-school/.

12 Adam Christopher Knotts, "Young People in Recovery from Substance Use Disorders: An Analysis of a Recovery High School's Impact on Student Academic Performance & Recovery Success," PhD diss., 2017.

13 Amy Yule and John Kelly, "Recovery High Schools May Be a Key Component of Youth Recovery Support Services," *American Journal of Drug and Alcohol Abuse* 44, no. 2 (2018): 141.

14 D. Paul Moberg and Andrew J. Finch, "Recovery High Schools: A Descriptive Study of School Programs and Students," *Journal of Groups in Addiction & Recovery* 2, no. 2–4 (2008): 128–161.

Chapter 20

1 Faces and Voices of Recovery, *Recovery Community Organization Toolkit,* January 2012, https://facesandvoicesofrecovery.org/arco/rco-toolkit/.

2 Beverly Haberle et al., "The Recovery Community Center: A New Model for Volunteer Peer Support to Promote Recovery," *Journal of Groups in Addiction & Recovery* 9, no. 3 (2014): 257–270.

3 Phillip Valentine, William White, and Pat Taylor, "The Recovery Community Organization: Toward a Definition," Selected Papers: William L. White, 2007, www.williamwhitepapers.com/papers.

4 Laudet and Humphreys, "Promoting Recovery in an Evolving Policy Context."

5 The largest proportion of people going to RCCs are unemployed men in their first year of recovery with primary opioid or alcohol problems and involved in the criminal justice system. John Kelly et al., "New Kid on the Block: An Investigation of the Physical, Operational, Personnel, and Service Characteristics of Recovery Community Centers in the United States," *Journal of Substance Abuse Treatment* 111 (2020): 1–10.

6 Kelly et al., "One-Stop Shopping for Recovery."

7 Sharon Reif et al., "Peer Recovery Support for Individuals with Substance Use Disorders: Assessing the Evidence," *Psychiatric Services* 65, no. 7 (2014): 853–861; and Bassuk et al., "Peer-Delivered Recovery Support Services for Addictions in the United States: A Systematic Review," *Journal of Substance Abuse Treatment* 63 (2016): 1–9.

8 Center for Substance Abuse Treatment, *What Are Peer Recovery Support Services?* HHS Publication No. (SMA) 09-4454 (Rockville, MD: Substance Abuse and Mental Health Services Administration, 2009).

9 Connecticut Community for Addiction Recovery, *Recovery Coach Academy Trainer's Manual,* January 2018.

10 New Hampshire Recovery Hub website: https://nhrecoveryhub.org/about-us.

11 Bassuk et al., "Peer-Delivered Recovery Support Services."

12 David Eddie et al., "Lived Experience in New Models of Care for Substance Use Disorder: A Systematic Review of Peer Recovery Support Services and Recovery Coaching," *Frontiers in Psychology* 10 (2019): 1052.

13 William White and Arthur C. Evans, "The Recovery Agenda: The Shared Role of Peers and Professionals," *Public Health Reviews* 35, no. 2 (2013): 4.

Chapter 21

1 According to Faces and Voices of Recovery (FAVOR), this messaging recommendation is based on public opinion research with members of the recovery community and the general public. FAVOR suggests that people in recovery, family members, and friends use this messaging style. FAVOR provides in-person and virtual "Our Stories Have Power" trainings. See https://facesandvoicesofrecovery.org/training/.

2 William White, "The New Recovery Advocacy Movement Basics," Selected
   Papers: William L. White, January 2016, www.williamwhitepapers.com
   /blog/2016/01/new-recovery-advocacy-movement-basics.html. For more on the
   New Recovery Advocacy Movement, see William L. White, *Let's Go Make Some
   History: Chronicles of the New Addiction Recovery Advocacy Movement* (Washington,
   DC: Johnson Institute Foundation, 2006).

3 Alliance for Addiction Payment Reform, "Addiction Recovery Medical Home
   Alternative Payment Model: Incentivizing Recovery, Not Relapse," 2019, https://
   incentivizerecovery.org/.

INDEX

ABOUT THE AUTHOR

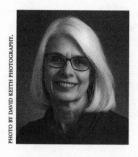

Author and public health professional Alison Jones Webb of Charlottesville, Virginia, is a passionate advocate for people in recovery from addictions. She has written extensively about issues related to recovery from addiction and harm reduction.

Webb, who holds master's degrees in public health (focusing on overdose prevention) from the University of New England and in economic history from The Johns Hopkins University, is a certified prevention specialist, trained recovery coach, Recovery Ambassador with Faces and Voices of Recovery (the nation's leading recovery advocacy organization), and a member of the Virginia Recovery Advocacy Project (a part of the national Recovery Advocacy Project's network of grassroots activists). She is president of the Maine Association of Recovery Residences and an active volunteer in numerous other recovery-related efforts.

Webb also has more than twenty years of experience in public speaking, policy development and advocacy, data-driven decision making, nonprofit strategic planning, community outreach and organizing, and linking community members with health care.

About North Atlantic Books

North Atlantic Books (NAB) is a 501(c)(3) nonprofit publisher committed to a bold exploration of the relationships between mind, body, spirit, culture, and nature. Founded in 1974, NAB aims to nurture a holistic view of the arts, sciences, humanities, and healing. To make a donation or to learn more about our books, authors, events, and newsletter, please visit www.northatlanticbooks.com.